Recent Advances in Spine Tumor Diagnosis and Treatment

Recent Advances in Spine Tumor Diagnosis and Treatment

Guest Editor

Jae Hwan Cho

MDPI

Basel • Beijing • Wuhan • Barcelona • Belgrade • Novi Sad • Cluj • Manchester

Guest Editor
Jae Hwan Cho
Department of Orthopedic
Surgery
University of Ulsan College
of Medicine
Seoul
Republic of Korea

Editorial Office
MDPI AG
Grosspeteranlage 5
4052 Basel, Switzerland

This is a reprint of the Special Issue, published open access by the journal *Journal of Clinical Medicine* (ISSN 2077-0383), freely accessible at: https://www.mdpi.com/journal/jcm/special_issues/M9W9WHFATM.

For citation purposes, cite each article independently as indicated on the article page online and as indicated below:

Lastname, A.A.; Lastname, B.B. Article Title. *Journal Name* **Year**, *Volume Number*, Page Range.

ISBN 978-3-7258-6662-5 (Hbk)
ISBN 978-3-7258-6663-2 (PDF)
https://doi.org/10.3390/books978-3-7258-6663-2

Contents

About the Editor

Jae Hwan Cho

Jae Hwan Cho is a Professor of Orthopedic Surgery at Asan Medical Center, University of Ulsan College of Medicine in Seoul, Korea. His clinical and academic work is centered around spine surgery, with broad interests that include spinal oncology, lumbar degenerative disease, and adult spinal deformity. Dr. Cho received his medical degree and completed his doctoral studies at Seoul National University College of Medicine.

Dr. Cho has authored more than 200 peer-reviewed publications and has presented extensively at major international scientific meetings, including ISSLS, EuroSpine, and IMAST. His research encompasses clinical decision-making in degenerative and oncologic spinal disease, optimization of surgical strategies, and outcome improvement across the cervical, thoracic, and lumbar spine.

In addition to his clinical and research activities, Dr. Cho contributes to academic leadership and collaborative scholarship. He serves as Deputy Editor of the *Asian Spine Journal* and holds active roles within the Korean Society of Spine Surgery and the Korean Society of Spine Tumor. Through his work, he remains committed to advancing evidence-based care, improving functional outcomes, and enhancing quality of life for patients with spinal disorders.

Preface

This Reprint brings together recent advances in the diagnosis, evaluation, and treatment of spinal tumors, an area that continues to grow in clinical relevance as survival improves for patients with systemic cancer. The purpose of assembling this collection was to provide a practical, evidence-based resource for clinicians who manage patients with metastatic involvement of the spine, primary spinal tumors, and treatment-related complications.

The scope of this Reprint reflects the rapidly evolving landscape of spine oncology. Several articles evaluate surgical and radiotherapeutic approaches for metastatic epidural spinal cord compression, addressing one of the most time critical oncologic emergencies. Other studies explore clinical issues arising from stereotactic body radiotherapy, including local control and vertebral compression fracture risk. Additional contributions examine prognostic and decision-making tools such as nutritional status indices, cervical instability scoring, Hounsfield unit-based bone quality assessment, and predictors of instrumentation failure. Emerging technologies are also represented through systematic reviews of artificial intelligence applications in prognosis estimation and imaging interpretation. A case-based report further illustrates rare complications encountered in real-world practice.

This Reprint is intended for spine surgeons, radiation and medical oncologists, radiologists, and all members of multidisciplinary teams caring for patients with spinal tumors. It is my hope that the enclosed work provides useful perspectives for treatment planning, highlights the importance of individualized care, and encourages continued inquiry into strategies that enhance functional outcomes and quality of life. I am grateful for the efforts of all contributors whose studies inform and advance the care of patients facing spinal tumors.

Jae Hwan Cho
Guest Editor

Journal of
Clinical Medicine

MDPI

Article

Clinical Outcomes of Surgery Versus Radiotherapy in Bilsky Grade 3 Metastatic Epidural Spinal Cord Compression

Kihyun Kwon , Sehan Park , Myeong Geun Song , Wan Soo Park, Chang Ju Hwang , Dong-Ho Lee and Jae Hwan Cho *

Department of Orthopedic Surgery, Asan Medical Center, University of Ulsan College of Medicine, Seoul 05505, Republic of Korea; 899835@naver.com (K.K.)
* Correspondence: spinecjh@gmail.com

Abstract

Background/Objectives: Surgery is generally recommended for higher Bilsky grade metastatic epidural spinal cord compression (MESCC); however, Bilsky grades 2–3 are often grouped together, leaving limited evidence for managing patients with Bilsky grade 3 MESCC who have not developed neurological deficits. This study aimed to evaluate whether, and when, surgery should be performed in Bilsky grade 3 MESCC. **Methods**: This retrospective cohort study included patients diagnosed with Bilsky grade 3 MESCC from January 2021 to January 2025. A total of 138 patients were assigned to a radiotherapy (RT) group (n = 54) or a surgery group (n = 65) based on initial treatment. Demographics, clinical data, treatment outcomes, and treatment modalities were analyzed. Logistic regression identified risk factors for local progression, motor recovery, and ambulatory outcomes. **Results**: Ninety-five patients (70.3%) initially presented with weakness. Among 30 patients diagnosed before neurological deficits, interval from diagnosis to onset was 17.2 ± 14 days. Local progression and survival rates did not significantly differ between the groups. Surgery was associated with a higher likelihood of motor recovery (odds ratio [OR] = 10.05, $p < 0.001$) and better ambulatory function (OR = 0.433, $p = 0.003$). Higher initial motor grade and lower Eastern Cooperative Oncology Group Performance Status scores were also linked to favorable ambulatory outcomes. **Conclusions**: In Bilsky grade 3 MESCC, the mean interval from diagnosis to weakness onset was 17.2 days. Local progression and survival did not differ between RT and surgery; however, surgery provided superior motor recovery and ambulatory outcomes. Early surgery may offer improved functional outcomes in Bilsky grade 3 MESCC.

Keywords: Bilsky grade 3; metastatic epidural spinal cord compression; radiation therapy; surgery; spinal metastases

1. Introduction

Metastatic epidural spinal cord compression (MESCC) imposes a substantial clinical burden on patients and often results in severe pain, neurological deficits, and multiple comorbidities [1]. Advances in radiotherapy (RT) have broadened treatment options for MESCC [2,3]. Lower Bilsky grade MESCC is typically managed effectively with RT alone [4], whereas surgery is generally recommended for higher-grade disease because of neurological risks [5].

Current guidelines, including the Neurologic, Oncologic, Mechanical, and Systemic (NOMS) framework and the Neurology-Stability-Epidural compression (NSE) assessment, do not differentiate between Bilsky grades 2 and 3 [6,7]. A recent study by Park et al. reported that RT yielded favorable local control in Bilsky grade 2 MESCC [8], prompting questions regarding appropriate management of Bilsky grade 3 MESCC. However, few studies have focused specifically on patients with Bilsky grade 3 MESCC. Delayed surgery has been associated with poorer recovery of ambulatory function in patients with neurological deficits [9], and prompt treatment can help minimize the duration of neurological compromise [10]. However, for patients without neurological deficits, evidence on whether and when surgery should be performed remains limited.

Therefore, we conducted a retrospective cohort study of patients with Bilsky grade 3 MESCC to identify the therapeutic window for patients presenting without neurological symptoms and to evaluate treatment approaches for local control and ambulatory outcomes.

2. Materials and Methods

2.1. Study Design and Patient Inclusion

After institutional review board approval (IRB: 2025-0812), we conducted a retrospective cohort study of patients diagnosed with Bilsky grade 3 MESCC between January 2021 and January 2025. We searched our institutional data warehouse for magnetic resonance imaging interpretations containing "Grade 3," "ESCC 3," "MESCC 3," or "Bilsky 3." All interpretations were made by board-certified radiologists specializing in musculoskeletal imaging. An experienced board-certified orthopedic surgeon subsequently reviewed all images and excluded patients with inconsistent interpretations. Additional exclusion criteria were (1) MESCC below the conus medullaris, (2) a follow-up period <3 months, and (3) insufficient clinical data. Patients who died before 3 months were included.

2.2. Data Collection and Outcome Evaluation

Demographic variables included age, sex, comorbidities such as diabetes mellitus (DM) and hypertension (HTN), and smoking status. We also collected data on primary tumor pathology, Eastern Cooperative Oncology Group Performance Status (ECOG), and ambulatory ability. Baseline ECOG was defined as the patient's usual functional activity prior to the onset of neurological deterioration, in order to reflect pre-morbid systemic condition rather than disability related to acute cord compression or pain. ECOG at presentation and after treatment was also recorded but was not used as the primary variable for analysis. ECOG assessed after neurological deterioration was not used for baseline comparison, as it was frequently influenced by acute motor weakness. For further analysis, primary tumor pathologies were categorized according to radiosensitivity into three groups: radiosensitive, radioresistant, and intermediate. This classification was based on prior literature [11]. Tumors known to be radiosensitive or radioresistant were assigned accordingly, and those not clearly belonging to either category were allocated to the intermediate group. Imaging data included tumor level, compression direction, presence of pathologic fracture, and Spine Instability Neoplastic Score (SINS). Treatment decisions after diagnosis of Bilsky grade 3 MESCC were reviewed, and patients initially treated with RT were classified into an RT group, whereas patients treated surgically were assigned to a surgery group. Decisions regarding initial treatment modality were reached through multidisciplinary consensus among oncologists, spine surgeons, and radiation oncologists. Treatment allocation incorporated several clinical factors, including baseline ECOG performance status, SINS, comorbidity burden, estimated life expectancy, prior radiotherapy to the involved level, anatomical feasibility of decompression and stabilization, and patient preference. Patients who were initially evaluated as potential surgical candidates but ultimately did not undergo surgery, due to systemic deterioration,

 https://doi.org/10.3390/jcm15010216

comorbidities, or preference, were analyzed in the radiotherapy group. Patients who did not receive any active treatment or received only chemotherapy were included in the dataset for descriptive purposes but were excluded from comparative analyses. Treatment modality information, including surgical approach and technique, RT modality, external beam radiation therapy (EBRT) or stereotactic body radiation therapy(SBRT), RT dosage per fraction, and total dosage, was collected.

Outcome measures included local progression, motor recovery, and ambulatory function. Local progression was defined as tumor progression occurring after treatment that required further intervention at the same anatomical level. This determination was made based on a combination of clinical symptoms and follow-up MRI findings. Motor strength was evaluated using the modified Medical Research Council (mMRC) scale; the lowest recorded strength was used for analysis. Improvement in the same myotome was considered recovery; unchanged strength was considered maintained, and decreased strength was considered worsened. Logistic regression analyses excluded patients who had maintained grade 5 motor strength throughout. Motor recovery was categorized as favorable, whereas maintained or worsened strength was classified as an adverse outcome. Ambulatory function was assessed by the ability to walk; preserved or restored walking ability was considered success, whereas loss of ambulation was considered failure. Post-treatment imaging was not performed at fixed intervals. Follow-up MRI was obtained when patients developed new or worsening symptoms, or when clinical reassessment raised concern for progression. This symptom-driven imaging approach was applied similarly in both the surgery and radiotherapy groups.

2.3. Statistical Analyses

Statistical analyses were performed using SPSS version 24 (IBM Corp., Chicago, IL, USA) and Python version 3.11.8 (statsmodels 0.13.5, scikit-learn 1.1.3). A two-sided p-value < 0.05 was considered statistically significant. Student's t test or Mann–Whitney U test was used for continuous variables, and the chi-square test was used for categorical variables. Logistic regression was used to identify risk factors for the outcomes. Kaplan–Meier survival analysis was performed to compare survival between the two groups.

3. Results

After applying the inclusion and exclusion criteria, 138 patients were included (Figure 1). Fifty-four patients (39.1%) received initial RT, and 65 (47.1%) underwent surgery. Five patients (3.6%) received chemotherapy, and 14 (10.1%) chose conservative management. Among the 95 patients (70.3%) who presented with weakness, 30 (31.6%) were diagnosed before weakness developed. The mean interval from diagnosis to onset of weakness was 17.2 ± 14 days (Figure 2 top). Although a few patients developed weakness after more than 40 days, most had an intervention window of less than 30 days once diagnosed with Bilsky grade 3 MESCC. Patients who initially presented with pain were treated within 15.5 ± 13.8 days (Figure 2 bottom). Two patients presented with pain alone and began RT 29 and 30 days after diagnosis, but later developed weakness.

https://doi.org/10.3390/jcm15010216

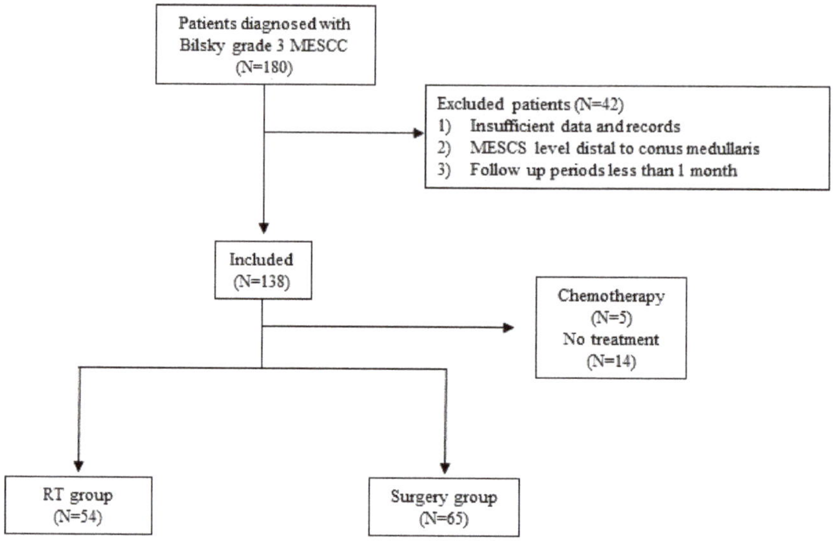

Figure 1. Flow chart of patient selection process.

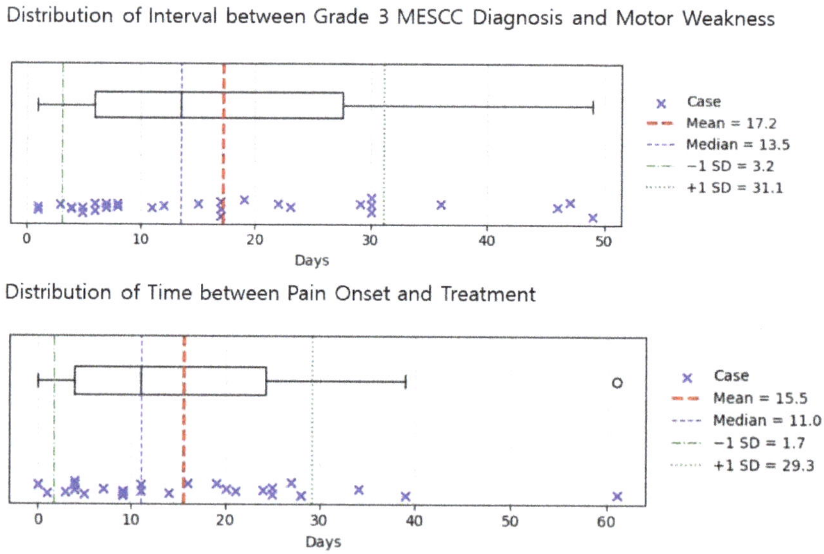

Figure 2. Distribution of the interval from diagnosis to onset of motor weakness (**top**) and the interval from pain onset to treatment initiation (**bottom**).

3.1. Comparison Between the RT and Surgery Groups

We compared patients treated with RT with those treated surgically (Table 1). Demographic characteristics were not significantly different between the groups. Initial symptoms varied, and weakness was more common as a presenting symptom in the surgery group. The average motor grade was also more severe in the surgery group than in the RT group. Other parameters, including the ECOG status, involved location, presence of pathologic fracture, direction of compression, and SINS, did not differ significantly. We examined reasons for selecting RT instead of surgery for patients presenting with weakness (Figure 3). In 36% of patients, surgical procedures and general anesthesia were not feasible.

https://doi.org/10.3390/jcm15010216

In 55% of patients, the surgical department elected not to perform surgery despite referral. Ten percent of patients had a favorable response to RT, and 4% declined surgery.

Table 1. Comparison of demographics between RT and Surgery group.

	RT Group (N = 54)	Surgery Group (N = 65)	*p*-Value
Patient demographics			
Age	61.62 (±11.86)	58.12 (±12.41)	0.124
Sex (M:F)	34:20	48:17	0.235
DM	8	12	0.615
HTN	20	13	0.208
Smoking	22	27	1.000
Pathology			0.301
Lung	17	16	
HCC	10	12	
RCC	2	5	
Breast cancer	2	3	
GI	6	10	
Hematologic	4	4	
GU	9	3	
OBGY	2	4	
Sarcoma	2	3	
Others	0	5	
Clinical symptoms			
ECOG	2.10 ± 1.22	2.12 ± 1.09	0.895
Initial symptoms			0.003 *
No symptom	2	0	
Pain	23	14	
Weakness	29	51	
Motor grade for patients with weakness	3.54 ± 1.72	2.90 ± 1.54	0.042 *
Image findings			
Involved location (Cervical:Thoracic:Multiple)	6:45:3	8:56:1	0.499
Pathologic fracture	24	42	0.063
Compression direction (Anterior:Posterior:Circumferential)	5:6:43	10:7:48	0.673
SINS	10.27 ± 3.23	11.08 ± 2.84	0.16

RT: Radiotherapy; M: Male; F: Female; DM: Diabetes Mellitus; HTN: Hypertension; HCC: Hepatocellular carcinoma; RCC: Renal cell carcinoma; GI: Gastrointestinal; GU: Genitourinary; OBGY: Obstetrics and gynecology; ECOG: Eastern Cooperative Oncology Group Performance Status; SINS: Spine Instability Neoplastic Score. * *p*-value < 0.05.

Table 2 presents the comparison of clinical outcomes between the groups. Motor recovery and ambulation recovery rates were significantly higher in the surgery group. More patients in this group demonstrated improved or stable motor strength, whereas a higher proportion of patients in the RT group experienced worsened motor strength after treatment. Local progression rate, survival duration, and complication rate did not differ significantly. Kaplan–Meier survival analysis showed no difference between the groups (Figure 4).

https://doi.org/10.3390/jcm15010216

Table 2. Outcome comparison between RT and Surgery group.

	RT Group (N = 54)	Surgery Group (N = 65)	*p*-Value
Motor recovery			<0.001 *
Improved	6	32	
Maintained	24	27	
Worsened	24	6	
Ambulation recovery			0.017 *
Success	21	40	
Failure	33	25	
Local progression	11(20.3%)	15 (23.1%)	0.825
Survival period	6.31 ± 6.01	7.55 ± 7.17	0.600
Complications	2	5	0.454

RT: Radiotherapy. * *p*-value < 0.05.

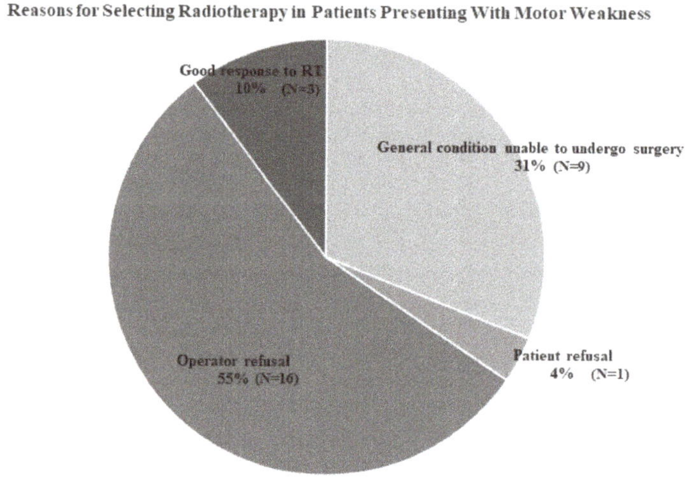

Figure 3. Pie chart illustrating the reasons for selecting radiotherapy over surgery in patients presenting with motor weakness.

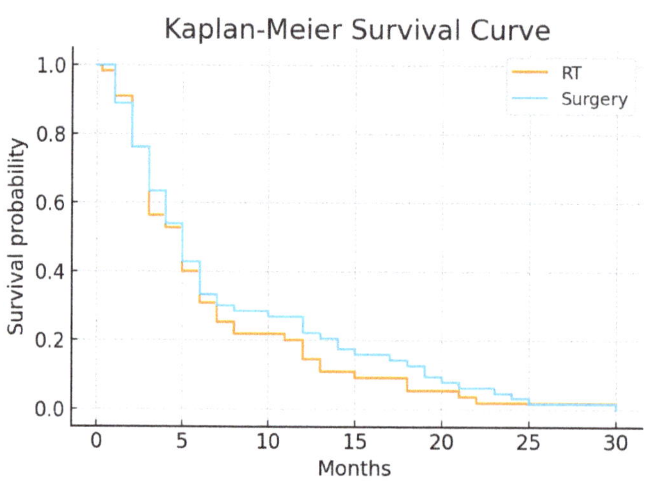

Figure 4. Kaplan–Meier survival curves comparing overall survival between the radiotherapy and surgery groups.

https://doi.org/10.3390/jcm15010216

To identify risk factors for local progression, we further analyzed patients according to specific approaches and RT modalities. Most patients in the surgery group underwent a posterior approach with laminectomy and fusion (Table 3). Among patients who received RT, 41.9% underwent SBRT, and 44.4% of patients initially treated with RT received SBRT. A relatively large proportion of patients did not undergo postoperative RT (n = 22, 33.8%). Most of these patients (n = 8, 36%) were unable to receive postoperative RT because their general condition deteriorated after surgery (Figure 5). A substantial number (n = 6, 27%) were lost to follow-up during transfers between departments or hospitals. Additionally, 23% of patients (n = 5) could not receive postoperative RT due to preoperative RT history.

Table 3. Treatment approaches and modes for both Surgery and RT patients.

	Patient Treated with Operation
Operation Approach	
Anterior	5 (7.7%)
Posterior	57 (88.6%)
Combined	3 (4.6%)
Operation type	
Laminectomy	2 (3%)
Laminectomy and fusion	59 (90.8%)
Corpectomy	4 (6.2%)
Postop RT	
Yes	43 (66.2%)
No	22 (33.8%)
RT type	
EBRT	25 (58.1%)
SBRT	18 (41.9%)
	Patient treated with Radiotherapy
RT type	
EBRT	30 (55.6%)
SBRT	24 (44.4%)

RT: Radiotherapy; EBRT: external beam radiation therapy; SBRT: stereotactic body radiation therapy.

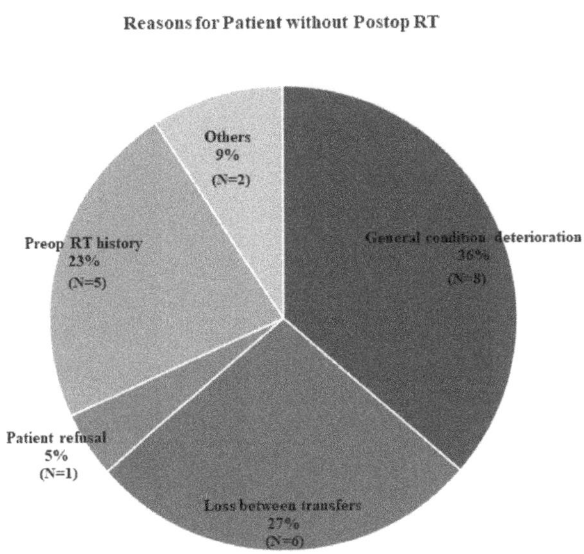

Figure 5. Pie chart illustrating the reasons why some patients did not receive postoperative radiotherapy after surgery.

https://doi.org/10.3390/jcm15010216

When stratified by tumor radiosensitivity, local progression, ambulatory recovery, and motor improvement were comparable among the sensitive, intermediate, and resistant groups. In RT-treated patients, outcomes were likewise similar across radiosensitivity categories, none reaching statistical significance (Supplementary Tables S1 and S2).

3.2. Risk Factor Analysis for Local Progression, Motor Recovery, and Ambulatory Outcomes

After subcategorization, we evaluated risk factors for local progression (Table 4). DM was a significant risk factor, with an odds ratio (OR) of 3.00 (95% confidence interval [CI] 1.07–8.40; $p = 0.04$). In the surgery group, postoperative RT showed a marginal protective effect (OR 0.32; $p = 0.06$). DM was also a risk factor in the RT group. The initial treatment modality (surgery vs. RT) did not significantly influence the risk of local progression. Multivariate analysis confirmed these findings, with postoperative RT maintaining marginal significance.

Table 4. Regression analysis of risk factors for local progression.

All Patients	Univariate OR (95% CI)	*p*-Value	Multivariate OR (95% CI)	*p*-Value
Age	0.99 (0.96–1.03)	0.73		
Sex (F)	0.60 (0.22–1.65)	0.32	—	—
DM	3.00 (1.07–8.40)	0.037 *	2.89	0.050 *
HTN	0.55 (0.19–1.61)	0.28	—	—
Smoking	1.06 (0.44–2.56)	0.89	—	—
Pathology	0.82 (0.39–1.73)	0.36	—	—
ECOG	0.99 (0.68–1.45)	0.96	—	—
Initial motor power	0.90 (0.69–1.17)	0.44	—	—
Tumor Location (Cervical, Thoracic, Multiple)	1.12 (0.79–1.59)	0.52	—	—
Pathologic Fx	1.00	0.09	—	—
Compression direction (Ant, post, circumferential)	1.00	0.33	—	—
SINS total score	0.98 (0.85–1.13)	0.81	—	—
Initial Tx (Surgery vs. RT)	1.17 (0.49–2.82)	0.72	—	—
RT modality (SBRT)	0.89 (0.35–2.23)	0.80	—	—
Surgery Group				
Age	0.99 (0.94–1.04)	0.64	—	—
Sex (F)	0.64 (0.16–2.63)	0.54	—	—
DM	1.91 (0.48–7.52)	0.36	—	—
HTN	0.49 (0.10–2.47)	0.39	—	—
Smoking	1.86 (CI 0.58–5.97)	0.29	—	—
ECOG	1.03 (0.60–1.75)	0.92	—	—
Initial motor grade	0.82 (0.56–1.20)	0.31	—	—
Tumor Location (Cervical, Thoracic, Multiple)	—	0.49	—	—
Pathologic Fx	1.12 (0.33–3.81)	0.85	—	—
Compression direction (Ant, post, circumferential)	—	0.13	—	—
SINS total	0.99 (0.81–1.21)	0.90	—	—
Postoperative RT	0.32 (0.10–1.06)	0.061 *	0.29 (0.08–1.03)	0.055 *
Surgery type	—	0.73	—	—

 https://doi.org/10.3390/jcm15010216

Table 4. *Cont.*

All Patients	Univariate OR (95% CI)	*p*-Value	Multivariate OR (95% CI)	*p*-Value
RT Group				
Age	1.003 (0.95–1.06)	0.92	—	—
Sex (F)	0.57 (0.13–2.47)	0.46	—	—
DM	5.57 (1.12–27.66)	0.036 **	5.44 (1.02–29.00)	0.047 **
HTN	0.63 (0.15–2.74)	0.54	—	—
Smoking	0.47 (0.11–2.03)	0.31	—	—
Pathology	—	0.21	—	—
ECOG	0.95 (0.55–1.64)	0.86	—	—
Tumor Location (Cervical, Thoracic, Multiple)	—	0.47	—	—
Pathologic Fx	0.76 (0.20–2.87)	0.68	—	—
Compression direction (Ant, post, circumferential)	—	0.67	—	—
SINS total	0.97 (0.79–1.19)	0.78	—	—
RT modality (SBRT)	0.66 (0.17–2.58)	0.55	—	—
Dose per Fraction	1.00 (0.994–1.006)	0.55	—	—
Total Radiation Dose	1.00 (0.997–1.014)	0.17	—	—

RT: Radiotherapy; F: Female; DM: Diabetes Mellitus; HTN: Hypertension; ECOG: Eastern Cooperative Oncology Group Performance Status; Fx: Fracture; SINS: Spine Instability Neoplastic Score; Tx: Treatment; SBRT: stereotactic body radiation therapy. * *p*-value near 0.05, ** *p*-value < 0.05.

Regression analysis for motor recovery was conducted (Table 5). Surgery as the initial treatment demonstrated a strong favorable association with recovery (OR = 9.82, 95% CI 3.49–27.67, $p < 0.001$). Higher SINS were linked to a greater likelihood of recovery (OR = 1.20, 95% CI 1.03–1.40, $p = 0.02$). However, in the multivariate analysis, only treatment modality remained significant (OR = 10.05, 95% CI 3.36–30.10, $p < 0.001$). Ambulatory outcomes were also analyzed (Table 6). Surgery as the initial treatment (OR = 4.33, 95% CI 1.66–11.29, $p = 0.003$) and higher initial motor power (OR = 1.57, 95% CI 1.12–2.19, $p = 0.01$) were significantly associated with better ambulation. Higher ECOG grades were associated with poorer outcomes (OR = 0.60, 95% CI 0.40–0.92, $p = 0.02$). Cervical metastasis showed a trend toward better outcomes than thoracic or multilevel metastases (OR = 0.26, 95% CI 0.07–1.07, $p = 0.05$), although this was not significant in the multivariate analysis.

Table 5. Regression analysis of risk factors for Motor recovery.

All Patients (N = 80)	Univariate OR (95% CI)	*p*-Value	Multivariate OR (95% CI)	*p*-Value
Age	1.11 (0.97–1.04)	0.812		
Sex (F)	1.00 (0.46–2.72)	0.950	—	—
DM	0.96 (0.32–2.85)	0.942		
HTN	0.56 (0.22–1.44)	0.23	—	—
Smoking	0.78 (0.34–1.80)	0.56	—	—
Pathology	—	0.71	—	—
ECOG	1.24 (0.86–1.80)	0.25	—	—
Initial motor power	1.12 (0.87–1.44)	0.39	—	—
Location (C/T/M)	0.38	0.14	—	—
Pathologic Fx	1.01 (0.43–2.36)	0.99	—	—
Compression direction (Ant, post, circumferential)	—	0.23	—	—
SINS total score	1.20 (1.03–1.40)	0.02 *	1.18 (0.99–1.40)	0.07
Initial Tx (Surgery)	9.82 (3.49–27.67)	<0.001 **	10.05 (3.36–30.10)	<0.001 **
RT modality (SBRT)	0.76 (0.31–1.86)	0.55	—	—

RT: Radiotherapy; F: Female; DM: Diabetes Mellitus; HTN: Hypertension; ECOG: Eastern Cooperative Oncology Group Performance Status; C; Cervical; T: Thoracic; M: Multiple; Fx: Fracture; SINS: Spine Instability Neoplastic Score; Tx: Treatment; SBRT: stereotactic body radiation therapy. * *p*-value < 0.05, ** *p*-value < 0.005.

 https://doi.org/10.3390/jcm15010216

Table 6. Regression analysis of risk factors for ambulation recovery.

All Patients	Univariate OR (95% CI)	p-Value	Multivariate OR (95% CI)	p-Value
Initial treatment Surgery vs. RT	2.33 (1.10–4.90)	0.03 *	4.33 (1.66–11.29)	0.003 **
ECOG	0.47 (0.33–0.68)	<0.001 **	0.60 (0.40–0.92)	0.02 *
Initial motor power	1.57 (1.21–1.99)	<0.001 **	1.57 (1.12–2.19)	0.01 **
Metastasis level Thoracic vs. Cervical	0.26 (0.07–1.07)	0.05 *	0.28 (0.07–1.16)	0.08
Metastasis level Multiple vs. Cervical	0.09 (0.01–1.60)	0.07	0.09 (0.01–1.56)	0.09

OR: Odds ratio; CI: Credible interval; RT: Radiotherapy; ECOG: Eastern Cooperative Oncology Group Performance Status. * p-value < 0.05, ** p-value < 0.005.

4. Discussion

In our study, we analyzed patients with Bilsky grade 3 MESCC. The average interval between diagnosis of Bilsky grade 3 MESCC and onset of weakness was 17.2 ± 14 days. Patients presenting with neurologic deficits were more often treated surgically. Local progression and survival rates did not differ between the groups; however, motor strength recovery and ambulatory function were superior in the surgery group. Treatment modality was not a risk factor for local progression, but it had a significant effect on motor strength recovery and ambulatory outcomes.

In our study, patients with Bilsky grade 3 appeared more vulnerable to neurological deficits. Among 138 included patients, 90 had motor weakness, and 60 of them showed weakness prior to diagnosis. Even in patients without clinical symptoms of neurological deficit, the safety margin was very short, averaging 17.2 days. Patients who presented with pain only were also treated within 30 days to remain free of neurological deterioration. These results differ from the finding that 67% of Bilsky grade 2 patients initially presented with pain [7]. However, prior work reported that paralysis severity was not associated with the degree of cord compression [12], our findings suggest that higher compression grades may carry a greater risk of paralysis. Therefore, we propose that patients diagnosed with Bilsky grade 3 MESCC should be considered for early surgical intervention.

Secondly, in our cohort, a substantial proportion of patients (25 of 29, 86.2%) were treated with RT rather than surgery because of comorbidities and the risk of deterioration in overall condition. Given that patients with higher Bilsky grades have poorer survival [11], previous studies have emphasized careful patient selection to limit surgical stress in frail individuals [13]. In our cohort, survival and complication rates were not significantly different between the two groups. Even among patients with limited life expectancy, quality of life should remain a key factor when considering a surgical intervention [14]. Therefore, if survival outcomes are comparable between surgery and RT, surgical treatment may be recommended more strongly. However, as this was a retrospective cohort study, patients in better general condition may have been more likely to receive surgery, whereas those in poorer condition may have been directed toward RT. A small number of patients who were initially considered for surgery but ultimately treated with radiotherapy due to clinical deterioration were included in the radiotherapy group (n = 3). Although this subgroup was very small relative to the overall cohort, its inclusion may still contribute to residual confounding, and this should be considered when interpreting the comparative results. Baseline ECOG performance status was comparable between the two groups. Nevertheless, ECOG alone may not fully capture differences in systemic fitness, and residual selection bias is likely to persist. Additional studies are needed to further clarify these observations.

https://doi.org/10.3390/jcm15010216

The local progression rate did not differ between the groups, and neither surgery nor RT was a risk factor for local progression. In our study, only DM was associated with local progression. Previous reports have shown that DM contributes to immune dysfunction, which may worsen outcomes in metastatic cancer, aligning with our findings [15–17]. However, the small sample size introduces the possibility of confounding factors that require further evaluation. Although postoperative RT demonstrated a marginally significant protective effect, this result is consistent with the findings of Hu et al. [2]. Despite the established importance of postoperative RT for improved outcomes, many patients were lost during intra- or inter-hospital transfers, preventing them from receiving postoperative RT. To reduce the risk of recurrence, enhanced communication across transfer settings is essential.

The SINS is recognized as an important determinant when selecting surgery or RT [18,19]. However, most patients with Bilsky grade 3 MESCC in our cohort had a high SINS, which limited its significance in the analysis. The radiation modality also did not significantly influence progression. Although SBRT showed a numerically lower rate of local progression compared with EBRT, this difference did not reach statistical significance. Wong et al. similarly reported no difference in local progression between EBRT and SBRT [20,21], which is consistent with our findings. Radiation dose per fraction was also not associated with local progression in our cohort, despite prior reports suggesting its importance [22]. This may reflect the small sample size of the SBRT subgroup and the consequent limited ability to adjust for confounders such as radiosensitivity, tumor biology, and prior RT exposure. Therefore, the absence of a statistically significant difference between SBRT and EBRT should be interpreted with caution. Accordingly, no definitive conclusions regarding the comparative efficacy of EBRT versus SBRT can be drawn from this dataset.

Motor strength and ambulatory recovery were superior in the surgery group. Although higher SINS values were associated with improved recovery in the univariate analysis, this association was not significant in the multivariate analysis. This finding likely reflects that patients with higher SINS values were more likely to undergo surgery, suggesting confounding between SINS values and treatment modality. When categorized by ambulatory function, ECOG score and initial motor power were significant predictors of recovery. Because ECOG performance status reflects ambulatory capacity, and motor grade is essential for ambulation, these results align with our expectations. Although surgery intuitively offers greater potential for motor and ambulatory improvement because direct spinal cord decompression is more effective than RT [23,24], few studies have evaluated these outcomes specifically in patients with Bilsky grade 3 MESCC.

Because patients with Bilsky grade 3 MESCC face a high risk of rapid neurologic deterioration, and given the superior functional outcomes observed with surgery along with comparable comorbidity profiles, survival rates, and local progression rates, we propose surgery as the preferred treatment for patients with or without weakness.

The main limitation of this study is its retrospective design, which prevents complete exclusion of selection bias in the treatment choice. In addition, the number of patients was too small for meaningful subgroup analyses or identification of additional risk factors. For instance, we could not differentiate tumor pathologies, although distinct pathologies may yield different outcomes. Variations in radiosensitivity based on primary pathology may substantially influence treatment results [25]. Hepatocellular carcinoma showed a higher local progression rate than other pathologies in our cohort, but the sample size (22 cases) was insufficient for statistical significance. Large, multi-center studies are necessary to obtain more comprehensive data on the relatively uncommon Bilsky grade 3 MESCC and to validate the findings of this study.

https://doi.org/10.3390/jcm15010216

5. Conclusions

In patients diagnosed with Bilsky grade 3 MESCC, the mean interval to weakness onset was 17.2 days. Local progression and survival did not differ between RT and surgery. Surgical treatment was associated with better motor recovery and ambulatory outcomes. Timely surgical intervention in Bilsky grade 3 MESCC may offer better functional results in appropriately selected patients. Further prospective studies are needed to validate these findings.

Supplementary Materials: The following supporting information can be downloaded at: https://www.mdpi.com/article/10.3390/jcm15010216/s1/.

Author Contributions: Conceptualization, J.H.C. and S.P.; Methodology, K.K. and S.P.; Software, K.K.; Validation, S.P. and J.H.C.; Formal Analysis, K.K.; Investigation, K.K.; Resources, J.H.C.; Data Curation, M.G.S., W.S.P., C.J.H., and D.-H.L.; Writing—Original Draft Preparation, K.K.; Writing—Review and Editing, S.P.; Visualization, K.K.; Supervision, J.H.C.; Project Administration, J.H.C. All authors have read and agreed to the published version of the manuscript.

Funding: This research received no external funding.

Institutional Review Board Statement: The study was conducted according to the guidelines of the Declaration of Helsinki, and approved by the Institutional Review Board of Asan Medical Center (2025-0812, approval date: 4 July 2025).

Informed Consent Statement: Patient consent was waived due to the retrospective nature of the study.

Data Availability Statement: The data presented in this study are available on request from the corresponding author due to ethical and institutional regulations, the data are not publicly available.

Acknowledgments: The authors have obtained permission to reproduce all copyrighted materials included in this manuscript, where applicable.

Conflicts of Interest: The authors declare no conflicts of interest.

Abbreviations

The following abbreviations are used in this manuscript:

MESCC	Metastatic epidural spinal cord compression
RT	Radiotherapy
SBRT	Stereotactic body radiation therapy
EBRT	External beam radiation therapy
DM	Diabetes mellitus
HTN	Hypertension
ECOG	Eastern Cooperative Oncology Group performance status
SINS	Spine Instability Neoplastic Score
mMRC	Modified Medical Research Council
OR	Odds ratio
CI	Confidence interval
IRB	Institutional review board

References

1. Van den Brande, R.; Cornips, E.M.; Peeters, M.; Ost, P.; Billiet, C.; Van de Kelft, E. Epidemiology of spinal metastases, metastatic epidural spinal cord compression and pathologic vertebral compression fractures in patients with solid tumors: A systematic review. *J. Bone Oncol.* **2022**, *35*, 100446. [CrossRef] [PubMed]
2. Hu, J.X.; Gong, Y.N.; Jiang, X.D.; Jiang, L.; Zhuang, H.Q.; Meng, N.; Liu, X.G.; Wei, F.; Liu, Z.J. Local Tumor Control for Metastatic Epidural Spinal Cord Compression Following Separation Surgery with Adjuvant CyberKnife Stereotactic Radiotherapy or Image-Guided Intensity-Modulated Radiotherapy. *World Neurosurg.* **2020**, *141*, e76–e85. [CrossRef]

3. Park, S.; Lee, D.H.; Hwang, C.J.; Cho, J.H. Spine surgery for metastatic spine cancer in the era of advanced radiation therapy. *Asian Spine J.* **2025**. [CrossRef]
4. Vavourakis, M.; Sakellariou, E.; Galanis, A.; Karampinas, P.; Zachariou, D.; Tsalimas, G.; Marougklianis, V.; Argyropoulou, E.; Rozis, M.; Kaspiris, A.; et al. Comprehensive Insights into Metastasis-Associated Spinal Cord Compression: Pathophysiology, Diagnosis, Treatment, and Prognosis: A State-of-the-Art Systematic Review. *J. Clin. Med.* **2024**, *13*, 3590. [CrossRef]
5. Laufer, I.; Rubin, D.G.; Lis, E.; Cox, B.W.; Stubblefield, M.D.; Yamada, Y.; Bilsky, M.H. The NOMS Framework: Approach to the Treatment of Spinal Metastatic Tumors. *Oncology* **2013**, *18*, 744–751. [CrossRef]
6. Di Perna, G.; Baldassarre, B.; Armocida, D.; De Marco, R.; Pesaresi, A.; Badellino, S.; Bozzaro, M.; Petrone, S.; Buffoni, L.; Sonetto, C.; et al. Application of the NSE score (Neurology-Stability-Epidural compression assessment) to establish the need for surgery in spinal metastases of elderly patients: A multicenter investigation. *Eur. Spine J.* **2024**, *33*, 4302–4315. [CrossRef] [PubMed]
7. Park, S.; Lee, D.H.; Hwang, C.J.; Jeong, G.; Choi, J.U.; Sohn, H.J.; Kim, S.; Kim, Y.J.; Cho, J.H. Treatment Approach for Bilsky Grade 2 Metastatic Epidural Spinal Cord Compression Based on Radiation Therapy Failure Risk. *Glob. Spine J.* **2025**, 21925682251359292. [CrossRef]
8. Park, S.; Park, J.W.; Park, J.H.; Lee, C.S.; Lee, D.H.; Hwang, C.J.; Yang, J.J.; Cho, J.H. Factors affecting the prognosis of recovery of motor power and ambulatory function after surgery for metastatic epidural spinal cord compression. *Neurosurg. Focus* **2022**, *53*, E11. [CrossRef]
9. Laufer, I.; Zuckerman, S.L.; Bird, J.E.; Bilsky, M.H.; Lazáry, Á.; Quraishi, N.A.; Fehlings, M.G.; Sciubba, D.M.; Shin, J.H.; Mesfin, A.; et al. Predicting Neurologic Recovery after Surgery in Patients with Deficits Secondary to MESCC: Systematic Review. *Spine* **2016**, *41*, S224–S230. [CrossRef]
10. Guo, L.; Xu, Q.; Ke, L.; Wu, Z.; Zeng, Z.; Chen, L.; Chen, Y.; Lu, L. The impact of radiosensitivity on clinical outcomes of spinal metastases treated with stereotactic body radiotherapy. *Cancer Med.* **2023**, *12*, 13279–13289. [CrossRef] [PubMed]
11. Bendfeldt, G.A.; Chanbour, H.; Chen, J.W.; Gangavarapu, L.S.; LaBarge, M.E.; Ahmed, M.; Jonzzon, S.; Roth, S.G.; Chotai, S.; Luo, L.Y.; et al. Does Low-Grade Versus High-Grade Bilsky Score Influence Local Recurrence and Overall Survival in Metastatic Spine Tumor Surgery? *Neurosurgery* **2023**, *93*, 1319–1330. [CrossRef]
12. Uei, H.; Tokuhashi, Y.; Maseda, M. Analysis of the Relationship Between the Epidural Spinal Cord Compression (ESCC) Scale and Paralysis Caused by Metastatic Spine Tumors. *Spine* **2018**, *43*, E448–E455. [CrossRef]
13. Murotani, K.; Fujibayashi, S.; Otsuki, B.; Shimizu, T.; Sono, T.; Onishi, E.; Kimura, H.; Tamaki, Y.; Tsubouchi, N.; Ota, M.; et al. Prognostic Factors after Surgical Treatment for Spinal Metastases. *Asian Spine J.* **2024**, *18*, 390–397. [CrossRef]
14. Dea, N.; Versteeg, A.L.; Sahgal, A.; Verlaan, J.J.; Charest-Morin, R.; Rhines, L.D.; Sciubba, D.M.; Schuster, J.M.; Weber, M.H.; Lazary, A.; et al. Metastatic Spine Disease: Should Patients with Short Life Expectancy Be Denied Surgical Care? An International Retrospective Cohort Study. *Neurosurgery* **2020**, *87*, 303–311. [CrossRef] [PubMed]
15. Leshem, Y.; Dolev, Y.; Siegelmann-Danieli, N.; Sharman Moser, S.; Apter, L.; Chodick, G.; Nikolaevski-Berlin, A.; Shamai, S.; Merimsky, O.; Wolf, I. Association between diabetes mellitus and reduced efficacy of pembrolizumab in non-small cell lung cancer. *Cancer* **2023**, *129*, 2789–2797. [CrossRef]
16. Brown, J.C.; Zhang, S.; Ou, F.S.; Venook, A.P.; Niedzwiecki, D.; Lenz, H.J.; Innocenti, F.; O'Neil, B.H.; Shaw, J.E.; Polite, B.N.; et al. Diabetes and Clinical Outcome in Patients with Metastatic Colorectal Cancer: CALGB 80405 (Alliance). *JNCI Cancer Spectr.* **2020**, *4*, pkz078. [CrossRef] [PubMed]
17. Rodrigues Mantuano, N.; Stanczak, M.A.; Oliveira, I.A.; Kirchhammer, N.; Filardy, A.A.; Monaco, G.; Santos, R.C.; Fonseca, A.C.; Fontes, M.; Bastos, C.S., Jr.; et al. Hyperglycemia Enhances Cancer Immune Evasion by Inducing Alternative Macrophage Polarization through Increased O-GlcNAcylation. *Cancer Immunol. Res.* **2020**, *8*, 1262–1272. [CrossRef]
18. Kildegaard, T.H.; Sabroe, D.; Wang, M.; Høy, K. How to select a treatment method for patients with potentially unstable metastatic vertebrae (spinal instability neoplastic score 7–12): A systematic review. *Asian Spine J.* **2025**. [CrossRef]
19. Serratrice, N.; Faddoul, J.; Tarabay, B.; Attieh, C.; Chalah, M.A.; Ayache, S.S.; Abi Lahoud, G.N. Ten Years After SINS: Role of Surgery and Radiotherapy in the Management of Patients with Vertebral Metastases. *Front. Oncol.* **2022**, *12*, 802595. [CrossRef]
20. Wong, H.C.Y.; Lee, S.F.; Chan, A.W.; Caini, S.; Hoskin, P.; Simone, C.B., 2nd; Johnstone, P.; van der Linden, Y.; van der Velden, J.M.; Martin, E.; et al. Stereotactic body radiation therapy versus conventional external beam radiotherapy for spinal metastases: A systematic review and meta-analysis of randomized controlled trials. *Radiother. Oncol.* **2023**, *189*, 109914. [CrossRef] [PubMed]
21. Ryu, S.; Deshmukh, S.; Timmerman, R.D.; Movsas, B.; Gerszten, P.; Yin, F.-F.; Dicker, A.; Abraham, C.D.; Zhong, J.; Shiao, S.L.; et al. Stereotactic Radiosurgery vs Conventional Radiotherapy for Localized Vertebral Metastases of the Spine: Phase 3 Results of NRG Oncology/RTOG 0631 Randomized Clinical Trial. *JAMA Oncol.* **2023**, *9*, 800–807. [CrossRef]
22. Kang, D.H.; Chang, B.S.; Kim, H.; Hong, S.H.; Chang, S.Y. Separation surgery followed by stereotactic ablative radiotherapy for metastatic epidural spinal cord compression: A systematic review and meta-analysis for local progression rate. *J. Bone Oncol.* **2022**, *36*, 100450. [CrossRef] [PubMed]

 https://doi.org/10.3390/jcm15010216

23. Patchell, R.A.; Tibbs, P.A.; Regine, W.F.; Payne, R.; Saris, S.; Kryscio, R.J.; Mohiuddin, M.; Young, B. Direct decompressive surgical resection in the treatment of spinal cord compression caused by metastatic cancer: A randomised trial. *Lancet* **2005**, *366*, 643–648. [CrossRef] [PubMed]
24. Quraishi, N.A.; Arealis, G.; Salem, K.M.; Purushothamdas, S.; Edwards, K.L.; Boszczyk, B.M. The surgical management of metastatic spinal tumors based on an Epidural Spinal Cord Compression (ESCC) scale. *Spine J.* **2015**, *15*, 1738–1743. [CrossRef] [PubMed]
25. Weber-Levine, C.; Jiang, K.; Al-Mistarehi, A.-H.; Welland, J.; Hersh, A.M.; Horowitz, M.A.; Davidar, A.D.; Sattari, S.A.; Redmond, K.J.; Lee, S.H.; et al. The role of combination surgery and radiotherapy in patients with metastatic spinal cord compression: What are the remaining grey areas? A systematic review. *Clin. Neurol. Neurosurg.* **2025**, *248*, 108632. [CrossRef]

https://doi.org/10.3390/jcm15010216

Journal of
Clinical Medicine

MDPI

Article

Local Control and Vertebral Compression Fractures After Stereotactic Body Radiotherapy for Spinal Metastases

Ha Un Kim, Jinhong Jung, Young Seok Kim, Yeon Joo Kim, Young Seob Shin and Su Ssan Kim *

Department of Radiation Oncology, Asan Medical Center, University of Ulsan College of Medicine, 88 Olympic-ro 43-gil, Songpa-gu, Seoul 05505, Republic of Korea; d210194@amc.seoul.kr (H.U.K.)
* Correspondence: watermountain@hanmail.net; Tel.: +82-2-3010-5680; Fax: +82-2-3010-6950

Abstract: Objectives: This study aimed to evaluate the efficacy and toxicity of stereotactic body radiotherapy (SBRT) for spinal metastases, focusing on pain control, local tumor control, and the incidence of vertebral compression fractures (VCF). **Materials and Methods:** We retrospectively analyzed 179 patients with 217 spinal metastatic lesions who underwent SBRT between July 2020 and April 2022. The prescribed doses for SBRT were 18 or 20 Gy for one fraction, ≥24 Gy for three fractions, ≥20 Gy for four fractions, and ≥25 Gy for five fractions. Patient-reported treatment response was evaluated 1–3 months after SBRT completion. Local recurrence was defined as failure within the radiotherapy field. Pain response, local progression-free survival (LPFS), and the incidence of painful VCF were assessed. Prognostic factors for LPFS and VCF risk factors were evaluated. **Results:** The overall pain response rate was 80.8%. LPFS rates were 90.6% at 1 year and 83.0% at 2 years. Lytic/mixed lesions and involvement of multiple segments were significant prognostic factors for reduced LPFS. The cumulative incidence of painful VCF was 8.7% at 1 year and 12.8% at 2 years. A biologically effective dose (BED_3) ≥104 Gy was the only significant risk factor for painful VCF. **Conclusions:** SBRT demonstrated high efficacy for pain and local tumor control in spinal metastases, with an acceptable VCF risk.

Keywords: spine; metastasis; stereotactic body radiotherapy; vertebral compression fracture

1. Introduction

Spinal metastasis is one of the frequent sites of tumor spread, occurring in approximately 50–70% of patients with cancer [1–3]. Among patients with spinal metastases, 20% exhibit symptoms that can result in serious complications, such as compression fractures or spinal cord compression [4]. The initial approach for managing patients with spinal metastases is to determine whether surgical intervention is required. For those not requiring surgery, conventional external beam radiotherapy (CRT) has been the standard treatment to relieve pain, improve or maintain neurological function, and achieve tumor control.

Recently, advances in targeted therapy, hormone-targeting drugs, and immune checkpoint inhibitors have improved long-term overall survival [5,6]. The prolonged survival has raised the importance of maintaining long-term local control of spinal metastases. In this context, stereotactic body radiotherapy (SBRT) offers several advantages over CRT, delivering high biologically effective doses (BED) of radiation to tumors while minimizing toxicities to surrounding normal tissues in a few fractions (typically 1–5). The efficacy of SBRT has been particularly notable in metastatic diseases with traditionally radioresistant histologies, such as renal cell carcinoma, hepatocellular carcinoma, and sarcoma [7,8]. Specifically in spinal metastases, SBRT has demonstrated superior outcomes compared to CRT, with high rates of tumor control (80–90%) and low rates of toxicity [9–11]. Large studies have reported overall and complete pain response rates of approximately 82% and 43.5%, respectively [12], and various SBRT doses and fractionation schemes were used in these studies. Large prospective studies have reported doses ranging from 16 or 20 Gy in a single fraction to 24 Gy in two fractions, 30 Gy in three fractions, or 35 Gy in five fractions [13].

However, vertebral compression fracture (VCF) is a potential late adverse effect of SBRT, causing pain and spinal instability, sometimes requiring stabilization or decompression. VCF rates are reported to be 6–14% [14]. Predictive factors for VCF have been identified including radiographic tumor features (e.g., lytic lesions or baseline VCF), patient characteristics (e.g., sex and age), and radiotherapy dose and fractionation (e.g., dose per fraction $\geq$ 20 Gy).

This study aims to assess patient-reported pain relief and evaluate the efficacy and incidence of VCF in patients with spinal metastases treated with SBRT at a large tertiary medical center in Korea.

2. Materials and Methods

We retrospectively reviewed the medical records of patients who underwent spinal SBRT at a single institution from July 2020 to April 2022. The inclusion criteria were as follows: (1) spinal metastasis confirmed by computed tomography (CT), magnetic resonance imaging (MRI), or positron emission tomography/CT (PET/CT); (2) age $\geq$ 18 years; and (3) Eastern Cooperative Oncology Group (ECOG) performance status of 0–2. Patients with previous surgery or radiotherapy to the involved vertebral region were excluded. Patient selection was based on our institutional guidelines, which recommend SBRT as primary treatment for patients with spinal metastases who have SINS scores < 7 (stable spine) and no or minimal neurological symptoms. In selected asymptomatic patients, SBRT was also offered to prevent progression that could lead to future pain or neurological compromise, to treat lesions with concerning radiographic features despite absence of symptoms, or according to institutional protocols recommending upfront SBRT for radioresistant histologies. Patients with SINS scores $\geq$ 13 or ESCC grade 3 requiring surgical intervention before radiotherapy were excluded from this study. Patients with multiple myeloma and other hematopoietic malignancies were also excluded, as these malignancies exhibit different radiosensitivity characteristics and patterns of spinal stability compared to solid tumors. A total of 179 patients were included in the analysis, with 217 treated lesions. Radiosensitive histology was defined as breast and prostate cancer. Radioresistant histology was defined as all other cancer types.

Before radiotherapy, the patients underwent a neurological examination and pain assessment. CT simulation was performed with a 2.5 mm slice thickness. Gross tumor volume was delineated using CT, MRI, or PET/CT, and clinical target volume was set by the radiation oncologist, considering tumor volume and organs at risk. Target volume doses were prescribed to be $\geq$95% of the radiotherapy dose. The selection of dose and fractionation was determined by a radiation oncologist, considering the characteristics of the spinal lesion and the dose constraints of the surrounding organs. The selection of dose and fractionation was determined by radiation oncologists based on several factors including distance to the spinal cord, tumor histology and size, ECOG, and history of previous radiotherapy. Based on these considerations, the schedule consisted of one to five fractions, with prescribed doses of 18 or 20 Gy for one fraction, $\geq$24 Gy for three fractions, $\geq$20 Gy for four fractions, and $\geq$25 Gy for five fractions. Simultaneous integrated boost (SIB) was permitted.

Patient-reported treatment response was evaluated 1–3 months after SBRT completion through medical records of follow-up visits and analgesic medications. Pain response was categorized as complete response (CR) (patients reporting being pain-free during follow-up visits), partial response (PR) (patients reporting feeling "less pain" compared to baseline, or documented reduction in analgesic medication dosage or frequency without increased pain), stable pain (patients reporting pain levels as "unchanged" or "the same" as baseline with stable medication requirements), or progressive pain (patients reporting worsening pain or requiring increased analgesic medication dosage). Only patients who provided clear, documented responses regarding their pain status during follow-up visits were included in the pain analysis. Patients without explicit pain-related reports or those with ambiguous responses were excluded from the pain assessment.

Radiologic response was assessed using CT, MRI, or PET/CT and evaluated according to the Response Evaluation Criteria in Solid Tumors (RECIST) ver. 1.1 and European Organization for Research and Treatment of Cancer PET criteria [15,16]. Local recurrence was defined as failure within the radiotherapy field. Local progression-free survival (LPFS) was calculated from the completion of radiotherapy to local recurrence.

Toxicity was evaluated according to the Common Terminology Criteria for Adverse Events (version 5.0). A painful VCF identified during a follow-up examination was defined as a new endplate fracture or progression of collapse deformity compared with the pre-SBRT imaging findings.

Survival curves for LPFS were constructed using the Kaplan–Meier method. All reported p-values are two-sided, and the significance level was set at 0.05 for all analyses. Cox and logistic regression analyses were used to determine the prognostic and risk factors for LRFS and painful VCF. Prognostic factors with p-values less than 0.1 were included in the multivariable analysis. All statistical analyses were performed using SPSS software, version 20.0 (IBM, Armonk, NY, USA).

3. Results

3.1. Characteristics of the Patients and Spinal Lesions

The baseline characteristics of the patients and lesions are summarized in Tables 1 and 2, respectively. The median age of all patients was 63 years, and the patients were predominantly male. The ECOG performance status was predominantly classified as 1. Among all treated lesions, 9.2% were cervical, 42.9% thoracic, 40.1% lumbar, and 7.8% sacral. The primary tumor histology included lung, prostate, gastrointestinal, breast, and others, in descending order of prevalence. Most lesions exhibited lytic characteristics (57.1%), were treated in a single segment (60.0%), and were documented to have pre-existing VCF based on MRI or CT scans before SBRT (25.8%). More than half of the lesions (76.5%) were symptomatic. Table 3 summarizes the dosimetry values and their associated characteristics. More than half of the lesions were treated with five fractions (66.4%) and SIB (58.5%). The median gross tumor volume and prescribed BED_{10} were 19.3 mL (range, 1.1–521.0) and 48.0 (range, 30.0–72.0), respectively.

Table 1. Patient characteristics.

Variables	Number of Patients (n = 179)
Age (years), median (range)	63 (29–86)
Sex	
Male	134 (74.9%)
Female	45 (25.1%)
ECOG	

Table 1. *Cont.*

Variables	Number of Patients (n = 179)
0	2 (1.1%)
1	145 (81.0%)
2	32 (17.9%)
BMI (kg/m^2), median (range)	23.5 (15.8–31.8)

Abbreviations: ECOG, Eastern Cooperative Oncology Group; BMI, body mass index.

Table 2. Lesion characteristics.

Variables	Number of Lesions (n = 217)
Bone agent use	
Yes	45 (20.7%)
No	172 (79.3%)
Histology	
Breast	7 (3.2%)
NSCLC	62 (28.6%)
Ureter	5 (2.3%)
Gastrointestinal	44 (20.3%)
Renal cell carcinoma	39 (18.0%)
Melanoma	1 (0.5%)
Prostate	46 (21.2%)
Gynecological	4 (1.8%)
Sarcoma	5 (2.3%)
Endocrinal	4 (1.8%)
Pain	
Yes	166 (76.5%)
No	51 (23.5%)
Spinal location	
Cervical	20 (9.2%)
Thoracic	93 (42.9%)
Lumbar	87 (40.1%)
Sacral	17 (7.8%)
Paraspinal extension	
Yes	48 (22.1%)
No	169 (77.9%)
Baseline vertebral compression fracture	
Yes	56 (25.8%)
No	161 (74.2%)
Bone lesion	
Lytic	126 (58.1%)
Blastic	62 (28.6%)
Mixed	29 (13.3%)
Number of segments treated	
Single	130 (60.0%)
Multiple (2–8)	87 (40.0%)

Abbreviations: NSCLC, non-small cell lung cancer.

Table 3. Dosimetric characteristics.

Characteristics	Number of Lesions (n = 217)
Fraction	
1	25 (11.5%)
3	8 (3.7%)
4	40 (18.4)
5	144 (66.4%)

Table 3. *Cont.*

Characteristics	Number of Lesions (n = 217)
GTV volume in cm^3, median (range)	19.3 (1.1–521.0)
Total prescription dose in Gy, median (range)	30.0 (16.0–40.0)
Fractional prescription dose, Gy, median (range)	6.5 (5.0–20.0)
Prescribed BED_{10}, Gy, median (range)	48.0 (30.0–72.0)
SIB	
Yes	127 (58.5%)
No	90 (41.5%)
Vertebral body dose maximum, median (range)	30 (0–40)
Vertebral body dose minimum, median (range)	24 (0–35)

Abbreviations: GTV, gross tumor volume; BED, biologically effective dose; SIB, simultaneous integrated boost.

3.2. Response to SBRT

The median follow-up period for the entire cohort was 15.3 months (range, 3.0–43.8). The outcomes of SBRT on the pain associated with each lesion are shown in Table 4. Among all lesions, 166 initially presenting with pain were evaluated for pain response to SBRT, excluding 51 lesions that did not present with pain. Sixty-one lesions (36.7%) achieved CR, and 96 lesions experienced PR.

Table 4. Pain assessment within three months of painful spinal metastases.

Response	Number of Painful Lesions at Baseline (n = 166)
Complete response	61 (36.7%)
Partial response	96 (57.8%)
Progressive pain	3 (1.8%)
Stable pain	6 (3.6%)

Among 217 lesions, 27 (12.4%) showed local recurrence at the irradiated sites. Of the 27 lesions with local recurrence, 13 (48.1%) occurred within the vertebral body, 2 (7.4%) within the epidural space, and 12 (44.4%) involved both sites. The cumulative incidence of local progression was 9.4% and 17.0% at 1 and 2 years, respectively (Figure 1A). Among these, five patients developed neurological deficits as a result of local tumor progression.

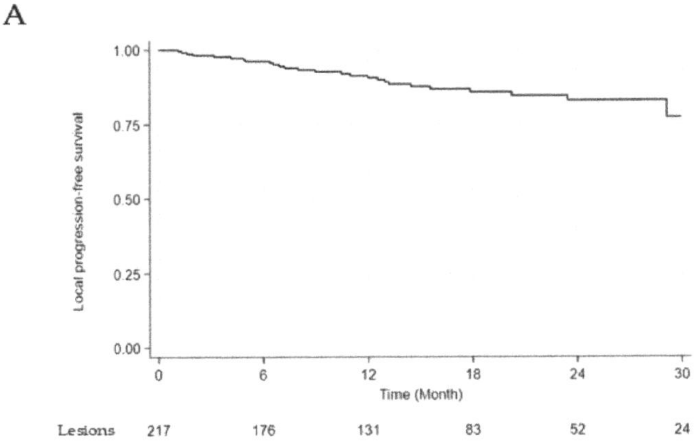

Figure 1. *Cont.*

B

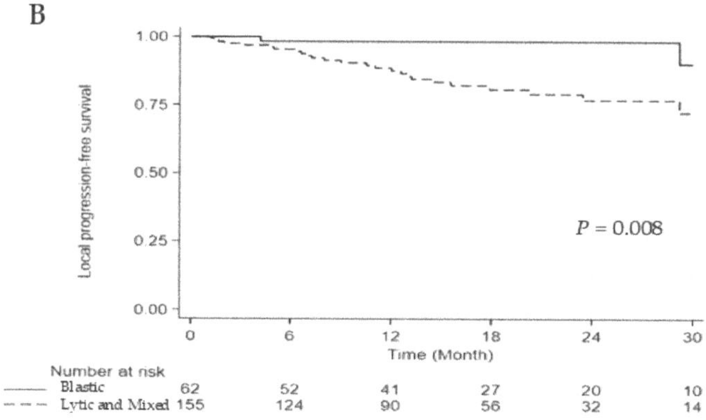

C

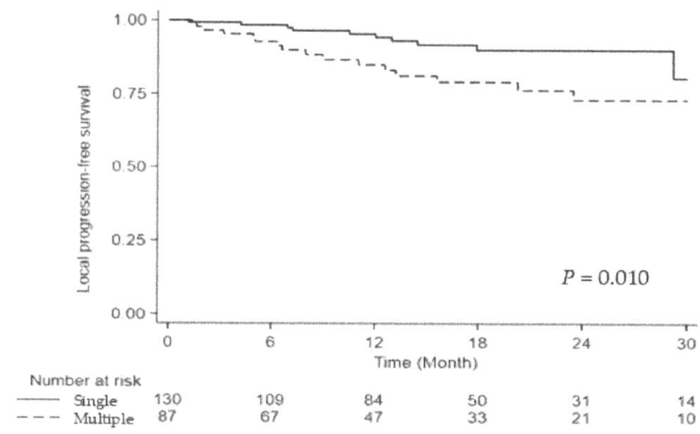

Figure 1. Kaplan–Meier Curve for (**A**) LPFS, (**B**) LPFS According to the Lesion Type, and (**C**) LPFS According to the Segment Number. Abbreviations: LPFS, local progression free survival.

The univariate and multivariate analyses for LPFS are discussed in Table 5. Compared with blastic lesions, lytic and mixed lesions were associated with significantly worse LPFS (hazard ratio [HR] 5.704, 95% confidence interval [CI] 1.349–24.119, $p = 0.018$), and involvement of multiple segments was also an adverse prognostic factor (HR 2.686, 95% CI 1.228–5.874, $p = 0.013$). Significant differences in LPFS were observed between blastic versus lytic and mixed lesions and single versus multiple segments (2-year LPFS: 98.3% vs. 76.8%, $p = 0.008$; 2-year LPFS: 90.0% vs. 73.0%, $p = 0.010$) (Figure 1B,C).

Table 5. Univariate and multivariate analysis of LPFS.

Variables	Univariate			Multivariate		
	HR	**95% CI**	***p*-Value**	**HR**	**95% CI**	***p*-Value**
Histology (radioresistant vs. radiosensitive)	1.879	0.710–4.975	0.204	-	-	-
Type of lesion (lytic/mixed vs. blastic)	5.670	1.341–23.967	0.018	5.704	1.349–24.119	0.018
Paraspinal extension (yes vs. no)	2.527	1.148–5.560	0.021	1.951	1.047–5.542	0.122
Fraction (single vs. multiple)	1.347	0.462–3.928	0.586	-	-	-

Table 5. *Cont.*

Variables	Univariate			Multivariate		
	HR	95% CI	*p*-Value	HR	95% CI	*p*-Value
Segment (multiple vs. single)	2.665	1.221–5.813	0.014	2.686	1.228–5.874	0.013
SIB (yes vs. no)	1.667	0.745–3.732	1.667	-	-	-
BED_{10} (<50Gy vs. ≥50Gy)	1.076	0.503–2.301	0.850	-	-	-

Values in the parentheses were set as the reference. Abbreviations: LPFS, local progression free survival; HR, hazard ratio; CI, confidence interval; SIB, simultaneous integrated boost; BED, biologically effective dose.

Acute toxicity was evaluated during and within 3 months of SBRT. Acute radiation-induced side effects were grade 1 or 2, including esophagitis (*n* = 2, 1.0%) and diarrhea (*n* = 2, 1.0%). No grade 3 or higher acute toxicities were reported.

3.3. Painful VCF

We analyzed the incidence of VCF, as shown in Figure 2. One hundred and seventy-nine lesions with a follow-up duration of at least six months were evaluated for the incidence of painful VCF. Twenty painful VCFs were noted among the 179 lesions. The cumulative incidence of painful VCF was 8.7% at 1 year and 12.8% at 2 years (Figure 2A). The incidence of painful VCF stratified by fractionation scheme is summarized in Table 6. The VCF rate for single fraction (*n* = 21) was 19.0% (95% CI: 7.7–40.0). For multi-fraction regimens, rates were 0% (95% CI: 0–39.0) for 3 fractions (*n* = 6), 15.2% (95% CI: 6.7–30.9) for 4 fractions (*n* = 33), and 9.2% (95% CI: 5.2–15.8) for 5 fractions (*n* = 119). While sample sizes were substantially uneven across groups, with 66.5% of evaluable lesions receiving 5 fractions, there was no statistically significant difference in VCF incidence among fractionation schemes ($p = 0.232$).

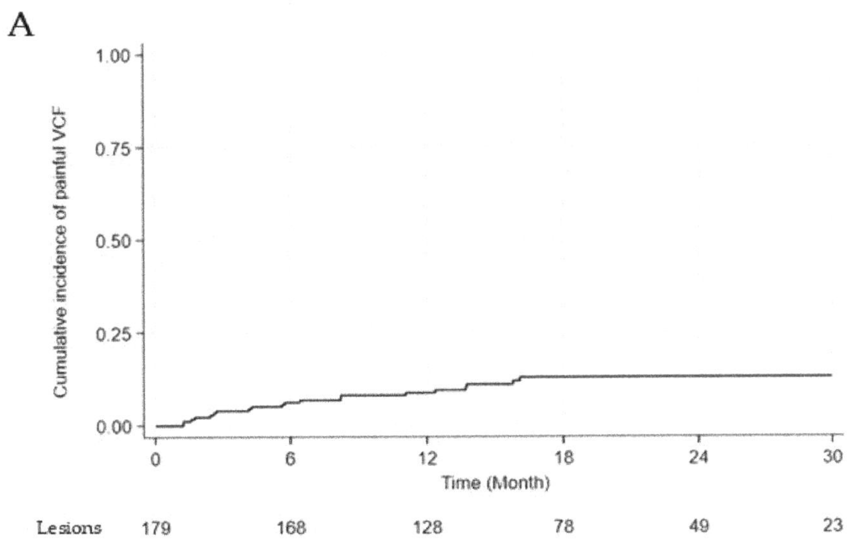

Figure 2. *Cont.*

B

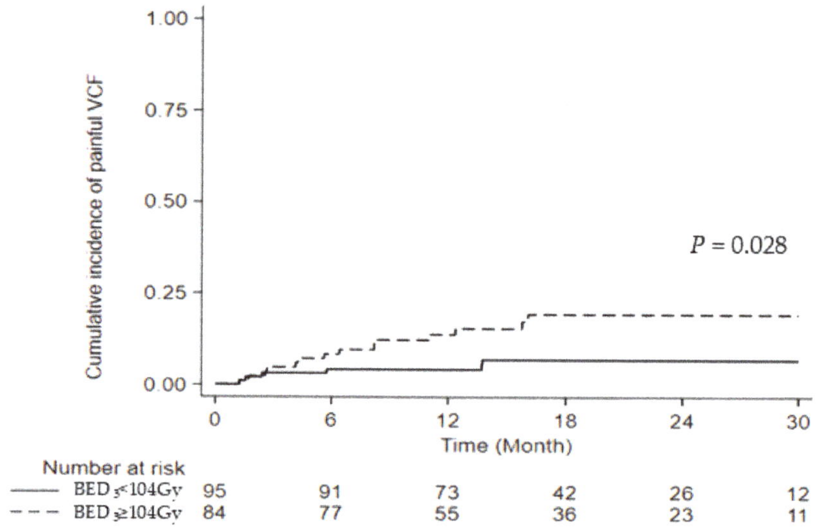

Figure 2. (**A**) Cumulative incidence of painful vertebral compression fractures (**B**) between BED_3 ≥104 Gy and <104 Gy. Abbreviations: VCF, vertebral compression fracture; BED, biologically effective dose.

Table 6. Painful vertebral compression fracture incidence by fractionation Scheme.

Fractionation	Total Number	Painful VCF Events (%)	95% CI
1 fraction	21	4 (19.0)	7.7–40.0
3 fractions	6	0 (0.0)	0.0–39.0
4 fractions	33	5 (15.2)	6.7–30.9
5 fractions	119	11 (9.2)	5.2–15.8

Abbreviations: VCF, vertebral compression fracture; CI, confidence interval.

Six lesions were treated with surgery for spinal stability, three lesions were managed with thoracolumbosacral orthosis, and 11 lesions were controlled with pain medications. Among those who underwent surgery, three patients experienced neurological deficits attributable to vertebral compression fractures. After univariate and multivariate analyses for painful VCF, BED_3 ≥104 Gy was the only significant risk factor (OR, 2.915; 95% CI, 1.045–8.132; $p = 0.041$) (Table 7). A significant difference was observed in the cumulative incidence of painful VCF between the BED_3 ≥104 Gy and BED_3 <104 Gy groups (2-year cumulative incidence of painful VCF: 19.3% vs. 6.9%, $p = 0.028$) (Figure 2A,B).

Table 7. Univariate and multivariate analyses of prognostic factors for painful vertebral compression fracture.

Variables	Univariate			Multivariate		
	OR	95% CI	*p*-Value	OR	95% CI	*p*-Value
Bone agent (no vs. yes)	1.560	0.524–4.644	0.425	-	-	-
BMI (<25 vs. ≥25)	2.997	0.841–10.673	0.090	2.830	0.775–10.332	0.115
Sex (female vs. male)	1.194	0.431–3.308	0.733	-	-	-

Table 7. *Cont.*

Variables	Univariate			Multivariate		
	OR	95% CI	*p*-Value	OR	95% CI	*p*-Value
Histology (radioresistant vs. radiosensitive)	1.032	0.322–3.305	0.957	-	-	-
Type of lesion (lytic/mixed vs. blastic)	4.500	1.006–20.120	0.049	4.212	0.825–19.173	0.063
Pre-existing VB collapse (yes vs. no)	2.123	0.808–5.058	0.127	-	-	-
Paraspinal extension (yes vs. no)	1.843	0.654–5.191	0.247	-	-	-
SINS class (II or greater vs. I)	1.957	0.758–5.049	0.165	-	-	-
Fraction (single vs. multiple)	2.088	0.625–6.972	0.231	-	-	-
SIB (yes vs. no)	1.656	0.605–4.533	0.326	-	-	-
Segment (multiple vs. single)	1.156	0.437–3.058	0.770	-	-	-
BED_3 (≥104Gy vs. <104 Gy)	2.967	1.085–8.115	0.034	2.915	1.045–8.132	0.041

Values in the parentheses were set as the reference. Abbreviations: OR, odds ratio; CI, confidence interval; BMI, body mass index; VB, vertebral body; SINS, Spinal Instability Neoplastic Score; SIB, simultaneous integrated boost; BED, biologically effective dose.

3.4. Subgroup Analysis

Subgroup analysis comparing symptomatic and asymptomatic lesions at baseline was performed to evaluate outcome differences by symptom status. Kaplan–Meier analysis showed a non-significant trend toward better local control in asymptomatic lesions ($p = 0.093$, log-rank test). One-year and two-year LPFS were 97.4% (95% CI, 82.8–99.6) and 92.9% (95% CI, 73.5–98.3) for asymptomatic lesions, versus 86.6% (95% CI, 79.4–91.4) and 80.0% (95% CI, 70.5–86.7) for symptomatic lesions. Local recurrence occurred in 3 of 51 asymptomatic lesions (5.9%) and 24 of 166 symptomatic lesions (14.5%). Among 179 lesions with ≥6 months of follow-up, painful VCF incidence was comparable between groups—4 of 45 (8.9%) versus 16 of 134 (11.9%) ($p = 0.574$).

3.5. Overall Survival

The median survival time was 17.3 months (range, 3.0–39.6), and the 1- and 2-year overall survival rates were 65.4% and 36.4%, respectively.

4. Discussion

This retrospective study demonstrated that SBRT is a highly effective treatment modality for managing pain and achieving local tumor control in patients with spinal metastases, with acceptable toxicity. The overall pain response rate to SBRT was 80.8%, which aligns with the evolving evidence base supporting SBRT for symptomatic spinal metastases. Early prospective evidence established SBRT efficacy, with Gerszen et al. reporting an overall pain response rate of 86% in one of the largest single-institution series of 500 cases [17]. Subsequently, higher-level evidence from the randomized controlled trials has confirmed SBRT's superiority. The landmark Canadian Cancer Trials Group Symptom Control 24 (CCTG SC.24) phase II/III clinical trial directly compared SBRT (24 Gy in 2 fractions) to CRT (20 Gy in 5 fractions) in 114 patients, demonstrating a complete pain response rate of 35% at 3 months with SBRT and establishing it as superior to conventional approaches for symptomatic disease [18]. A recent systematic review and meta-analysis by Guninski et al., conducted as part of the 2024 ESTRO practice guideline development, synthesized data from multiple studies and confirmed overall and complete pain response rates of approximately 83% and 36.5%, respectively, establishing contemporary benchmarks for SBRT efficacy [12]. Collectively, these data support SBRT as the preferred treatment modality for painful spinal metastases, and our results corroborate these findings in a real-world clinical setting.

Despite 75.6% of the lesions being classified as radioresistant, our study showed LPFS rates of 90.6% at 1 year and 83.0% at 2 years, consistent with previous studies reporting high tumor control rates (80–90%) with SBRT. These results compare favorably with CRT outcomes, with multiple studies now establishing SBRT's superiority for local control. The comparative study by Zeng et al. reported significantly lower local failure rates with SBRT versus CRT: 6.1% versus 28.4% at 12 months and 14.8% versus 35.6% at 24 months ($p < 0.001$) in a mature comparative analysis [19]. The CCTG SC.24 randomized trial similarly demonstrated improved local control with SBRT in their head-to-head comparison [18]. Our observed local recurrence rates of 9.4% at 1 year and 17.0% at 2 years with SBRT align with these findings and fall within the range reported by the systematic review by Guckenberger et al., which synthesized available evidence and reported local control rates of 80–95% at 1–2 years with SBRT, substantially higher than historical CRT [20]. However, several population-specific factors warrant consideration when interpreting these outcomes. The histologic composition of our cohort—mainly lung, prostate, and gastrointestinal cancers—may differ from other series, affecting the generalizability of local control estimates. The pronounced male predominance (74.9%), largely due to prostate and lung cancers, could have influenced lesion characteristics and treatment responses, as osteoblastic metastases from prostate cancer typically show better local control. In addition, the limited median overall survival (17.3 months) introduces competing mortality risk, whereby late recurrences may remain undetected. These factors should be considered when comparing our results with other studies. Optimal dose-fractionation for spinal SBRT remains an area of active investigation, with emerging evidence supporting higher biologically effective doses. The 2024 ESTRO clinical practice guideline, based on comprehensive systematic review, recommends a BED_{10} exceeding 50 Gy for durable local control, equivalent to a single fraction of 18 Gy or 30 Gy in three fractions [20]. This recommendation is supported by the randomized phase III trial by Zelefsky et al., which compared single-fraction 24 Gy versus fractionated 27 Gy in three sessions for oligometastatic disease, including 56% with spinal metastases, and demonstrated superior local control with the higher single-dose approach [21]. Long-term data from the SABR-COMET trial further support the efficacy of ablative doses in oligometastatic settings [13].

However, our analysis did not identify a significant dose–response relationship (no significant difference in LPFS between $BED_{10} \geq 50$ Gy and <50 Gy groups). This discrepancy warrants interpretation in the context of our population characteristics. First, our patient cohort included a higher proportion of multiple segments treatments (40.0% vs. single segment), which have been independently associated with reduced local control regardless of dose. Second, other factors, such as tumor histology or concurrent systemic therapies, may influence local control independent of the radiation dose. Additionally, the heterogeneity in the fractionation schedules used in our cohort might have affected the BED calculations and subsequent analysis. Further investigation into these potential confounding factors is warranted to better understand the dose–response relationship in this setting and to optimize SBRT regimens for individual patients. Our analysis identified lytic/mixed lesion characteristics and the involvement of multiple segments as significant prognostic factors for reduced LPFS. Similarly, Guckenberger et al. reported that treating >1 vertebra with SBRT correlated with poor local control ($p = 0.04$; HR, 0.62) in 387 spinal metastases [22]. Osteolytic lesions are known to exhibit more aggressive clinical features than osteoblastic lesions, often causing bone destruction and leading to mechanical instability of the spine. When we analyzed the histologies of lytic, mixed, and blastic lesions, more than half of the blastic lesions had primary tumors in the prostate and breast, while the lytic and mixed lesions were observed in the lung, gastrointestinal tract, and kidney. This heterogeneity in histology might have been attributed to the differences in local control.

Our subgroup analysis suggested modest differences in treatment outcomes according to baseline symptom status. Asymptomatic lesions showed marginally better local control than symptomatic lesions, with 2-year LPFS rates of 92.9% versus 80.0% ($p = 0.093$) and lower recurrence rates (5.9% vs. 14.5%). Although not statistically significant, this trend suggests that earlier intervention before symptom onset may be beneficial in carefully selected patients. The comparable incidence of painful VCF (8.9% vs. 11.9%, $p = 0.574$) indicates that prophylactic SBRT does not increase fracture risk. These findings support selective SBRT for asymptomatic lesions, particularly in patients with radioresistant histology or progressive disease despite systemic therapy, while underscoring the need for prospective validation.

Although the toxicity of SBRT for spinal metastases is generally considered acceptable, VCF is the most common adverse event, often resulting in significant pain and spinal deformity. Higher radiation doses can improve local control, but they increase the risk of VCFs, particularly with single-fraction schedules such as 1×24 Gy. We observed cumulative incidences of painful VCF of 8.7% at 1 year and 12.8% at 2 years, falling toward the lower end of the 6–14% range reported in the literature [14]. Several treatment-related factors may account for this relatively favorable toxicity outcome. Our predominant use of multi-fraction regimens likely allowed normal tissue repair between fractions. Additionally, bone-modifying agents were used in 20.7% of patients, which may have provided skeletal protection, particularly among high-risk individuals. Third, SIB was applied in 58.5% of lesions, potentially reducing vertebral body dose by concentrating radiation within the gross tumor volume. However, several potential sources of bias should be considered. The pronounced male predominance (74.9%), largely due to prostate (21.2%) and lung cancers (28.6%), may have attenuated the observed VCF incidence, as female sex is a known risk factor owing to lower bone mineral density and estrogen deficiency. Moreover, the limited median OS of 17.3 months introduces competing mortality risk, whereby late VCFs may remain undetected, likely leading to underestimation of the true cumulative incidence, particularly in longer-surviving populations.

Multiple risk factors for VCF following SBRT have been identified, including patient-related factors (SINS score, baseline fracture, lytic lesions, female sex) and treatment-related factors (dose per fraction, total dose) [14,19,20,22]. The 2024 ESTRO guideline confirmed dose per fraction ≥ 20 Gy as a significant predictor alongside patient-specific factors [20]. Our finding that $BED_3 \geq 104$ Gy was the only significant risk factor for painful VCF (HR 2.915, 95% CI 1.045–8.132, $p = 0.041$) aligns with prior dose-dependent VCF risk studies. The lack of association with other commonly reported risk factors may reflect our predominantly multi-fraction approach (88.5% received ≥ 3 fractions) and male-predominant population (74.9%). These findings underscore the importance of balancing tumor control against VCF risk through appropriate dose-fractionation selection.

Our study observed low rates of acute toxicity, with only grade 1–2 esophagitis and diarrhea reported in 2% of the cases. Therefore, SBRT can be a safe and effective treatment for patients with spinal metastases.

This study had several limitations. First, pain response was evaluated retrospectively from chart review rather than prospectively using standardized instruments such as the Brief Pain Inventory or Visual Analog Scale. Although we included only patients with clearly documented pain responses, the subjective nature of clinical records and inter-physician variability may have introduced inconsistencies. Pain assessment based on patient recall during follow-up may also be prone to bias. Moreover, the 1–3-month post-SBRT window, while clinically relevant, may not capture the full trajectory of pain improvement or late recurrence. Despite these limitations, our approach reflects real-world practice and provides meaningful insight into treatment efficacy. Second, the retrospective design carries inherent risks of selection bias and incomplete data capture, particularly for toxicity outcomes that may be underreported in routine clinical documentation. Third, several population-specific factors limit the generalizability of our findings. The marked male predominance (74.9%), largely due to high proportions of prostate and lung cancers, may have influenced lesion characteristics and the observed VCF incidence. The limited median OS of 17.3 months also introduces competing mortality risk, potentially leading to under-detection of late local recurrences and VCFs. In addition, the heterogeneous tumor histology in our cohort complicates direct comparison with other series. Future studies with more balanced populations and longer follow-up are needed. Fourth, imaging surveillance was not standardized, and some patients lacked pre- and post-SBRT MRI, which may have affected the accuracy of response and VCF assessment. Fifth, the marked attrition in patients at risk from 1 to 2 years in our Kaplan–Meier analyses may reduce the precision of long-term estimates and introduce survivor bias, as patients remaining at 2 years likely represent a more favorable subset. Accordingly, 2-year outcomes should be interpreted with caution, whereas 1-year estimates may better reflect the overall cohort. Sixth, our VCF risk factor analysis ($n = 20$ events) carries a potential risk of overfitting. To mitigate this, we restricted multivariable analysis to covariates with $p < 0.1$ in univariate testing, emphasized effect sizes over p-values, and included only biologically plausible variables. Validation in larger cohorts is warranted.

Despite these limitations, this study provides real-world evidence supporting the efficacy and safety of SBRT for spinal metastases in a large, consecutive patient cohort treated with contemporary techniques and dose-fractionation schemes.

We expect future studies to further investigate the prognostic factors for LPFS and risk factors for VCF, especially based on primary tumor histology. Our study demonstrated that SBRT is an effective and well-tolerated treatment for spinal metastases in terms of pain and local tumor control.

5. Conclusions

In this retrospective study, we evaluated the outcomes of SBRT in spinal metastases. SBRT emerges as an effective treatment for spinal metastases, achieving high rates of pain relief, local tumor control, and an acceptable risk of vertebral compression fractures.

Author Contributions: Conceptualization: S.S.K.; Investigation and methodology: H.U.K., J.J., Y.S.K., Y.J.K. and Y.S.S.; Writing the original draft: H.U.K.; Writing the review and editing: S.S.K. All authors have read and agreed to the published version of the manuscript.

Funding: This research received no external funding.

Institutional Review Board Statement: This study was approved by the Institutional Review Board at Asan Medical Center (IRB No.2024-0831, dated 2024-07-01), and informed consent was not required.

Informed Consent Statement: Patient consent was waived due to the retrospective nature of the study and the analysis used anonymous clinical data.

Data Availability Statement: Data supporting the findings of this study are available from the corresponding author upon reasonable request.

Conflicts of Interest: The authors have no conflicts of interest to declare.

References

1. National Collaborating Centre for Cancer (UK). National Institute for Health and Care Excellence: Guidelines. In *Metastatic Spinal Cord Compression: Diagnosis and Management of Patients at Risk of or with Metastatic Spinal Cord Compression;* National Collaborating Centre for Cancer: Cardiff, UK, 2008.
2. Perrin, R.G.; Laxton, A.W. Metastatic spine disease: Epidemiology, pathophysiology, and evaluation of patients. *Neurosurg. Clin. N. Am.* **2004**, *15*, 365–373. [CrossRef] [PubMed]
3. Harel, R.; Angelov, L. Spine metastases: Current treatments and future directions. *Eur. J. Cancer* **2010**, *46*, 2696–2707. [CrossRef] [PubMed]
4. Nater, A.; Martin, A.R.; Sahgal, A.; Choi, D.; Fehlings, M.G. Symptomatic spinal metastasis: A systematic literature review of the preoperative prognostic factors for survival, neurological, functional and quality of life in surgically treated patients and methodological recommendations for prognostic studies. *PLoS ONE* **2017**, *12*, e0171507. [CrossRef] [PubMed]
5. van den Bulk, J.; Verdegaal, E.M.; de Miranda, N.F. Cancer immunotherapy: Broadening the scope of targetable tumours. *Open Biol.* **2018**, *8*, 180037. [CrossRef]
6. Mok, T.; Camidge, D.R.; Gadgeel, S.M.; Rosell, R.; Dziadziuszko, R.; Kim, D.W.; Pérol, M.; Ou, S.I.; Ahn, J.S.; Shaw, A.T.; et al. Updated overall survival and final progression-free survival data for patients with treatment-naive advanced ALK-positive non-small-cell lung cancer in the ALEX study. *Ann. Oncol.* **2020**, *31*, 1056–1064. [CrossRef]
7. Altoos, B.; Amini, A.; Yacoub, M.; Bourlon, M.T.; Kessler, E.E.; Flaig, T.W.; Fisher, C.M.; Kavanagh, B.D.; Lam, E.T.; Karam, S.D. Local Control Rates of Metastatic Renal Cell Carcinoma (RCC) to Thoracic, Abdominal, and Soft Tissue Lesions Using Stereotactic Body Radiotherapy (SBRT). *Radiat. Oncol.* **2015**, *10*, 218. [CrossRef]
8. Singh, R.; Konrad, A.; Roubil, J.G.; Jenkins, J.; Davis, J.; Austin Vargo, J.; Gogineni, E.; Sharma, S. Improved local control following dose-escalated stereotactic ablative radiation therapy (SABR) for metastatic sarcomas: An international multi-institutional experience. *Radiother. Oncol.* **2024**, *190*, 110020. [CrossRef]
9. Redmond, K.J.; Sciubba, D.; Khan, M.; Gui, C.; Lo, S.L.; Gokaslan, Z.L.; Leaf, B.; Kleinberg, L.; Grimm, J.; Ye, X.; et al. A Phase 2 Study of Post-Operative Stereotactic Body Radiation Therapy (SBRT) for Solid Tumor Spine Metastases. *Int. J. Radiat. Oncol. Biol. Phys.* **2020**, *106*, 261–268. [CrossRef]
10. Sahgal, A.; Myrehaug, S.D.; Siva, S.; Masucci, L.; Foote, M.C.; Brundage, M.; Butler, J.; Chow, E.; Fehlings, M.G.; Gabos, Z.; et al. CCTG SC.24/TROG 17.06: A Randomized Phase II/III Study Comparing 24Gy in 2 Stereotactic Body Radiotherapy (SBRT) Fractions Versus 20Gy in 5 Conventional Palliative Radiotherapy (CRT) Fractions for Patients with Painful Spinal Metastases. *Int. J. Radiat. Oncol. Biol. Phys.* **2020**, *108*, 1397–1398. [CrossRef]
11. Sprave, T.; Verma, V.; Förster, R.; Schlampp, I.; Bruckner, T.; Bostel, T.; Welte, S.E.; Tonndorf-Martini, E.; Nicolay, N.H.; Debus, J.; et al. Randomized phase II trial evaluating pain response in patients with spinal metastases following stereotactic body radiotherapy versus three-dimensional conformal radiotherapy. *Radiother. Oncol.* **2018**, *128*, 274–282. [CrossRef]
12. Guninski, R.S.; Cuccia, F.; Alongi, F.; Andratschke, N.; Belka, C.; Bellut, D.; Dahele, M.; Josipovic, M.; Kroese, T.E.; Mancosu, P.; et al. Efficacy and safety of SBRT for spine metastases: A systematic review and meta-analysis for preparation of an ESTRO practice guideline. *Radiother. Oncol.* **2024**, *190*, 109969. [CrossRef]
13. Palma, D.A.; Olson, R.; Harrow, S.; Gaede, S.; Louie, A.V.; Haasbeek, C.; Mulroy, L.; Lock, M.; Rodrigues, G.B.; Yaremko, B.P.; et al. Stereotactic Ablative Radiotherapy for the Comprehensive Treatment of Oligometastatic Cancers: Long-Term Results of the SABR-COMET Phase II Randomized Trial. *J. Clin. Oncol.* **2020**, *38*, 2830–2838. [CrossRef]
14. Sahgal, A.; Atenafu, E.G.; Chao, S.; Al-Omair, A.; Boehling, N.; Balagamwala, E.H.; Cunha, M.; Thibault, I.; Angelov, L.; Brown, P.; et al. Vertebral compression fracture after spine stereotactic body radiotherapy: A multi-institutional analysis with a focus on radiation dose and the spinal instability neoplastic score. *J. Clin. Oncol.* **2013**, *31*, 3426–3431. [CrossRef]
15. Therasse, P.; Arbuck, S.G.; Eisenhauer, E.A.; Wanders, J.; Kaplan, R.S.; Rubinstein, L.; Verweij, J.; Van Glabbeke, M.; van Oosterom, A.T.; Christian, M.C.; et al. New guidelines to evaluate the response to treatment in solid tumors. European Organization for Research and Treatment of Cancer, National Cancer Institute of the United States, National Cancer Institute of Canada. *J. Natl. Cancer Inst.* **2000**, *92*, 205–216. [CrossRef] [PubMed]
16. Wahl, R.L.; Jacene, H.; Kasamon, Y.; Lodge, M.A. From RECIST to PERCIST: Evolving Considerations for PET response criteria in solid tumors. *J. Nucl. Med.* **2009**, *50* (Suppl. S1), 122s–150s. [CrossRef] [PubMed]
17. Gerszten, P.C.; Burton, S.A.; Ozhasoglu, C.; Welch, W.C. Radiosurgery for spinal metastases: Clinical experience in 500 cases from a single institution. *Spine* **2007**, *32*, 193–199. [CrossRef] [PubMed]
18. Sahgal, A.; Myrehaug, S.D.; Siva, S.; Masucci, G.L.; Maralani, P.J.; Brundage, M.; Butler, J.; Chow, E.; Fehlings, M.G.; Foote, M.; et al. Stereotactic body radiotherapy versus conventional external beam radiotherapy in patients with painful spinal metastases: An open-label, multicentre, randomised, controlled, phase 2/3 trial. *Lancet Oncol.* **2021**, *22*, 1023–1033. [CrossRef]
19. Zeng, K.L.; Myrehaug, S.; Soliman, H.; Husain, Z.A.; Tseng, C.L.; Detsky, J.; Ruschin, M.; Atenafu, E.G.; Witiw, C.D.; Larouche, J.; et al. Mature Local Control and Reirradiation Rates Comparing Spine Stereotactic Body Radiation Therapy with Conventional Palliative External Beam Radiation Therapy. *Int. J. Radiat. Oncol. Biol. Phys.* **2022**, *114*, 293–300. [CrossRef]

20. Guckenberger, M.; Andratschke, N.; Belka, C.; Bellut, D.; Cuccia, F.; Dahele, M.; Guninski, R.S.; Josipovic, M.; Mancosu, P.; Minniti, G.; et al. ESTRO clinical practice guideline: Stereotactic body radiotherapy for spine metastases. *Radiother. Oncol.* **2024**, *190*, 109966. [CrossRef]
21. Zelefsky, M.J.; Yamada, Y.; Greco, C.; Lis, E.; Schöder, H.; Lobaugh, S.; Zhang, Z.; Braunstein, S.; Bilsky, M.H.; Powell, S.N.; et al. Phase 3 Multi-Center, Prospective, Randomized Trial Comparing Single-Dose 24 Gy Radiation Therapy to a 3-Fraction SBRT Regimen in the Treatment of Oligometastatic Cancer. *Int. J. Radiat. Oncol. Biol. Phys.* **2021**, *110*, 672–679. [CrossRef]
22. Guckenberger, M.; Mantel, F.; Gerszten, P.C.; Flickinger, J.C.; Sahgal, A.; Létourneau, D.; Grills, I.S.; Jawad, M.; Fahim, D.K.; Shin, J.H.; et al. Safety and efficacy of stereotactic body radiotherapy as primary treatment for vertebral metastases: A multi-institutional analysis. *Radiat. Oncol.* **2014**, *9*, 226. [CrossRef]

Journal of
Clinical Medicine

MDPI

Article

Instrumentation-Related Complications Following Nonfusion Posterior Fixation in Patients with Metastatic Spinal Tumors: Incidence and Risk Factors

Yunjin Nam [1], Jin-Sung Park [2], Dong-Ho Kang [2], Chong-Suh Lee [3], Seung Woo Suh [1] and Se-Jun Park [2,*]

[1] Department of Orthopedic Surgery, Korea University Guro Hospital, Seoul 08308, Republic of Korea
[2] Department of Orthopedic Surgery, Samsung Medical Center, Seoul 06351, Republic of Korea
[3] Department of Orthopedic Surgery, Haeundae Bumin Hospital, Busan 48094, Republic of Korea
* Correspondence: sejunos@gmail.com; Tel.: +82-2-3410-1583

Abstract: Background/Objectives: Previous studies have reported satisfactory outcomes and low rates of instrumentation-related complications (IRCs) following nonfusion posterior fixation in patients with metastatic spinal tumors (MSTs). However, to adequately assess the longevity and durability of nonfusion instrumentation in patients with longer life expectancy, an extended follow-up period is essential. This study aims to evaluate the incidence of and risk factors for IRCs in patients with MSTs who underwent nonfusion posterior fixation and had radiographic follow-up data available for at least one year postoperatively. **Methods**: Consecutive data were collected from patients who underwent pedicle screw-based posterior fixation without fusion for MSTs in the thoracic and/or lumbar region from 2005 to 2018. The IRCs included screw loosening, screw pull-out, and metal breakage. The IRC-free survival and related factors were analyzed by Kaplan–Meier survivorship analysis with the log-rank test within a minimum follow-up period of one year. A multivariate analysis was performed using a Cox proportional-hazards regression model. **Results**: In total, 61 patients were included. The mean follow-up period was 28.3 months (range: 12.0–102.6 months). There were 27 cases (44.2%) of IRCs, including 22 cases of screw loosening, four cases of screw pull-out, and one case of rod breakage, at an average of 9.6 months (range: 1.0–38.1 months). The median IRC-free survival was 38.1 months (range: 1.0–102.6 months). Only three patients experienced pain aggravation with IRCs. No revision surgery was performed. A multivariate analysis identified that fixation length was a risk factor for IRCs (odds ratio: 0.358, 95% confidence interval: 0.114–0.888; $p = 0.027$). **Conclusions**: IRCs are frequent but mostly asymptomatic after nonfusion posterior fixation in patients with MSTs followed up for at least one year. Overall, the IRC-free survival was long enough considering the patient survival. Fixation length was a significant risk factor for IRCs regardless of MST location.

Keywords: metastatic spinal tumor; posterior fixation; nonfusion; instrumentation related complications; risk factors; survival analysis

1. Introduction

As the overall survival profile of cancer patients improves with continued advancements in medical treatment, the survival of patients with metastatic spinal tumors (MSTs) is also increasing [1]. Considering that the natural course of untreated MSTs would be unfavorable with time, those patients may experience pain or neurologic deficits related to MSTs [2,3]. Surgical treatment has been adopted more frequently than ever before to treat or prevent these morbidities in patients with MSTs [4]. Stabilization and/or decompression are the most popular surgical procedures included in palliative therapy plans [2].

Spinal fusion has been frequently paired with instrumentation to increase construct longevity and avoid late failures of instrumentation such as screw loosening, screw pull-out, or metal breakage [5,6]. In many patients with MSTs, however, the fusion procedure is difficult to complete due to a lack of adequate fusion bed or the individual's poor general condition. Additionally, fusion is difficult to achieve because of the effects of perioperative radiotherapy, chemotherapy, steroid use, and malnutrition [7]. Patients with MSTs usually have a relatively short life expectancy, which might not be long enough to achieve solid bony fusion [4]. For these reasons, spinal instrumentation without fusion has been considered in the management of MSTs.

Recent studies have reported favorable outcomes and low rates of instrumentation-related complications (IRCs) following nonfusion instrumentation in patients with MSTs [7–9]. However, many of these studies were limited by relatively short follow-up durations, making it difficult to assess the long-term durability of nonfusion constructs. Additionally, radiographic confirmation of instrumentation status at final follow-up was not consistently described. Evidence regarding IRC-free survival and associated risk factors in patients undergoing nonfusion surgery remains limited, particularly in those with longer life expectancy.

The current study aims to investigate the incidence of and risk factors for IRCs after posterior fixation without fusion in patients with MSTs. To evaluate long-term construct durability, we included a relatively large cohort of patients whose radiographic follow-up was available for at least 12 months after surgery.

2. Materials and Methods

2.1. Study Design

This study was a single-center, retrospective study performed using medical records. A total of 278 patients underwent surgical treatment for MSTs between 2005 and 2018. The main reasons for surgery in this group were severe axial pain with or without radiating pain or neurologic deficit. Decisions about whether to pursue surgical treatment and regarding which surgical option were made following a full discussion amongst the spine tumor board composed of medical oncologists, radiation oncologists, and spine surgeons.

To ensure consistency in the surgical technique analyzed, we first limited the cohort to those with thoracic or lumbar MSTs treated using pedicle screw fixation. This anatomical restriction excluded 51 patients with cervical or sacral lesions. Among the remaining 227 patients, 75 patients survived for more than one year based on their date of death or last follow-up visit. Among these, only those with radiographic follow-up—either plain radiographs or computed tomography (CT) scans—available at 12 months postoperatively were included.

CT imaging was not routinely performed but was included if chest or abdominopelvic CT scans taken for oncologic purposes included the operated spinal levels. Based on this criterion, 14 patients without appropriate imaging at the 12-month mark were excluded, resulting in a final cohort of 61 patients.

2.2. Surgical Procedures

The surgeries were performed by five spine surgeons at a single institute. All surgeries were performed using pedicle screw-based posterior fixation without any fusion procedures. The type of surgical procedure was determined by the spine tumor board by considering several factors, such as the main symptom of patients, the primary tumor site, and the location and extent of MSTs. For this study, we classified the surgical procedures chosen into three categories: posterior fixation without decompression, posterior fixation with laminectomy, and posterior fixation with debulking. Although the surgical procedures were determined variously by the surgeons, only posterior fixation was usually performed when radiographic instability was observed and mechanical pain was the main symptom without prominent neural compromise. In such cases, both open and percutaneous approaches were used. The choice between them was primarily guided by tumor location and anatomical accessibility: open fixation was preferred for thoracic lesions, whereas percutaneous fixation was more common for thoracolumbar junction and lumbar levels. For those with acute or subacute neurologic deficits with evidence of tumor invasion to the spinal canal, posterior fixation with laminectomy or debulking procedures were conducted. Debulking was performed via an anterior or posterior approach in patients with more favorable primary tumors and who were thought to be able to tolerate the aggressive surgery. When completing vertebrectomy during debulking surgery, the vertebral body was replaced by bone cement alone or bone cement within a mesh cage.

2.3. Outcome Measures

The main outcomes in this study were IRCs, which included screw loosening, screw pull-out, and metal breakage (Figure 1). IRCs were determined based on follow-up imaging at or beyond 12 months postoperatively using either plain radiography or CT imaging. Routine radiographic surveillance was conducted at approximately 3, 6, and 12 months postoperatively, followed by annual imaging. As in previous research, screw loosening was defined as the presence of a radiolucent zone measuring more than 1 mm surrounding the screw on the plain radiograph or CT scan [10]. Screw pull-out was defined as a 5° or greater change in the angle formed by the screw direction and upper endplate. Metal breakage was defined as any discontinuities in the implants. All imaging assessments were performed independently by one spine surgeon and one radiologist. Discrepancies were resolved by consensus or, when unresolved, based on the radiologist's interpretation.

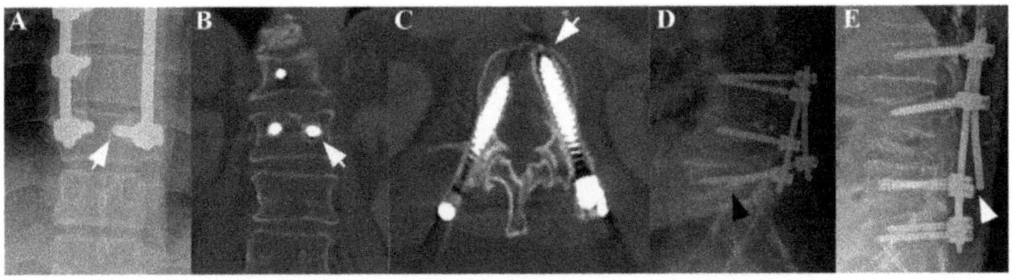

Figure 1. A plain anteroposterior (AP) radiograph (**A**) and coronal (**B**) and axial (**C**) CT scans of a patient subjected to posterior fixation showing radiological signs of screw loosening, indicated by the white arrows. Separately, plain lateral radiographs of a patient subjected to posterior fixation showing radiological signs of screw pull-out ((**D**), black arrowhead) and rod breakage ((**E**), white arrowhead).

When IRCs were observed during follow-up, an assessment of whether the pain was aggravated or not around the time of IRC identification was completed.

Risk factors for IRCs were evaluated according to the following variables: sex, age (<60 vs. ≥60 years), body mass index (<18.5, 18.5–24.9, or ≥25.0 kg/m^2), primary tumor site, number of vertebrae with metastases (1, 2, or ≥3 vertebrae), Spinal Instability Neoplasm Score criteria (stable, potentially unstable, or unstable) [11], location of metastases (at or above T10 vs. below T10), history of radiotherapy, location of the lowest instrumented vertebra (LIV) (at or above T10 vs. below T10), preoperative and postoperative Eastern Cooperative Oncology Group (ECOG) scale (0–2 vs. 3–4), type of surgical procedure (posterior fixation only, posterior fixation with laminectomy, or posterior fixation with debulking procedure), fixation length [number of instrumented vertebrae without metastases

(<3 vs. ≥3)] [12], screw density [number of pedicle screws per number of pedicles within the instrumented level (<0.67 or ≥0.67)] [13], and fixation method (open vs. percutaneous).

The presence or absence of metastases in each vertebra was primarily determined by magnetic resonance imaging (MRI), which served as the main diagnostic modality for evaluating tumor involvement.

2.4. Statistics

For univariate analysis, the presumed risk factors were compared in terms of IRC-free survival between patients with and without IRCs using Kaplan–Meier survivorship analysis with the log-rank test. Using the variables found to be significant with *p*-values of less than 0.05 during univariate analysis, a multivariate analysis was performed using a Cox proportional-hazards regression model. A forward stepwise procedure was adopted for the multivariate analysis. The statistical analysis was performed using the Statistical Package for the Social Sciences software program version 25.0.0 (IBM Corp., Armonk, NY, USA). A *p*-value of less than 0.05 was considered to be statistically significant.

3. Results

The study cohort consisted of 61 patients (37 men and 24 women, mean age of 61.7 years). The demographic and clinical data are described in Table 1.

Table 1. Demographic data of patients.

Variable	Value
Sex	
Male	37 (60.7%)
Female	24 (39.3%)
Age; mean ± SD, range (years)	61.7 ± 10.5, 31–83
<60	22 (36.1%)
≥60	39 (63.9%)
Body mass index (kg/m^2)	
<18.5	1 (0%)
18.5–24.9	38 (62.3%)
≥25	22 (37.7%)
Primary tumor site	
Lung	14 (23.0%)
Kidney	12 (19.7%)
Breast	8 (13.1%)
Liver	6 (9.8%)
Prostate	5 (8.2%)
Thyroid	4 (6.6%)
Colorectal	2 (3.3%)
Miscellaneous	10 (16.4%)
Number of involved vertebral bodies	
1	49 (80.3%)
2	7 (11.5%)
≥3	5 (8.2%)
SINS criteria *	
Stable	2 (3.3%)
Potential unstable	52 (85.2%)
Unstable	7 (11.5%)
Location of metastases	
At or above T10	27 (44.3%)
Below T10	34 (55.7%)

Table 1. *Cont.*

Variable	Value
History of radiotherapy	
Yes	55 (90.2%)
No	6 (9.8%)
Preoperative ECOG scale	
0–2	40 (65.6%)
3–4	21 (34.4%)
Postoperative ECOG scale	
0–2	54 (88.5%)
3–4	7 (11.5%)
Location of the LIV	
At or above T10	23 (37.7%)
Below T10	38 (62.3%)
Type of surgical procedure	
Posterior fixation only	19 (31.1%)
Posterior fixation with laminectomy	25 (41.0%)
Posterior fixation with debulking procedure	17 (27.9%)
Fixation length †	
<3	35 (57.4%)
≥3	26 (42.6%)
Screw density	
<0.67	24 (39.3%)
≥0.67	37 (60.7%)
Fixation method	
Open	46 (75.4%)
Percutaneous	15 (24.6%)

SD, standard deviation; SINS, spinal instability neoplastic score; ECOG, Eastern Cooperative Oncology Group; LIV, lowest instrumented vertebra. * SINS 0–6 represents stable, 7–12 potential unstable, and 13–18 unstable. † number of instrumented vertebrae without metastases.

There were no statistically significant differences in sex (p = 0.726) or age group (p = 0.266) between the included patients (n = 61) and those excluded due to insufficient follow-up, which was defined as either death within one year or absence of radiographic imaging at 12 months (n = 166). However, the distribution of primary tumor types showed a statistically significant difference (p < 0.001), suggesting that tumor biology may have influenced patient survival or follow-up availability. Additionally, no statistically significant differences were observed in sex (p = 1.000), age group (p = 0.250), or primary tumor type distribution (p = 0.634) between the included patients (n = 61) and those specifically excluded due to lack of imaging despite surviving longer than one year postoperatively (n = 14), indicating that radiographic loss to follow-up among long-term survivors was unlikely to have introduced meaningful selection bias.

The mean follow-up duration was 28.3 months (range: 12.0–102.6 months). At the point of final follow-up, 29 patients remained alive. The median overall survival after surgery was 35.6 months (95% CI, 21.2–50.0 months). Twenty-seven of these patients (44.1%) experienced IRCs at a mean of 9.6 months after surgery (range: 1.0–38.1 months). IRCs occurred less than one year after surgery in 19 cases and more than one year after surgery in eight cases. The most common IRC was screw loosening (n = 22 cases). The others included four cases of screw pull-out and one case of rod breakage. There were no cases characterized by screw breakage. Two cases of IRCs (one of screw loosening, one of screw pull-out) were accompanied by vertebral body fracture. Of these 27 patients with IRCs, only three patients (two with screw loosening, one with screw pull-out) experienced pain aggravation related to their respective IRCs. A patient with screw loosening accompanied by vertebral body fracture underwent cement augmentation. No revision surgeries were performed to address any of the IRCs.

The risk factors related to IRCs were analyzed using the log-rank test of the Kaplan–Meier survivorship analysis (Table 2).

Table 2. Factors related to IRCs by log-rank test of Kaplan–Meier survivorship analysis.

Variable	No. of Patients	No. of Patients with IRCs	*p*-Value
Sex			0.733
Male	37	16 (43.2%)	
Female	24	11 (45.8%)	
Age (years)			0.279
<60	22	8 (35.4%)	
≥60	39	19 (48.7%)	
Body mass index (kg/m^2)			0.777
<18.5	1	0 (0%)	
18.5–24.9	38	17 (44.7%)	
≥25	22	10 (45.4%)	
Primary tumor site			0.506
Lung	14	5 (35.7%)	
Kidney	12	6 (50.0%)	
Breast	8	2 (25.0%)	
Liver	6	2 (33.3%)	
Prostate	5	2 (40.0%)	
Thyroid	4	3 (75.0%)	
Colorectal	2	2 (100%)	
Miscellaneous	10	5 (50.0%)	
Number of involved vertebral bodies			0.992
1	49	22 (44.9%)	
2	7	3 (42.9%)	
≥3	5	2 (40.0%)	
SINS criteria †			0.325
Stable	2	0 (0%)	
Potential unstable	52	25 (48.1%)	
Unstable	7	2 (28.6%)	
Location of metastases			0.544
At or above T10	27	11 (40.7%)	
Below T10	34	16 (47.1%)	
History of radiotherapy			0.042 *
Yes	55	27 (49.1%)	
No	6	0 (0%)	
Preoperative ECOG scale			0.374
0–2	40	16 (40.0%)	
3–4	21	11 (52.4%)	
Postoperative ECOG scale			0.100
0–2	54	22 (40.7%)	
3–4	7	5 (71.4%)	
Location of the LIV			0.210
At or above T10	23	8 (34.8%)	
Below T10	38	19 (50.0%)	
Type of surgical procedure			0.073
Posterior fixation only	19	12 (63.2%)	
Posterior fixation with laminectomy	25	10 (40.0%)	
Posterior fixation with debulking procedure	17	5 (29.4%)	

Table 2. *Cont.*

Variable	No. of Patients	No. of Patients with IRCs	p-Value
Fixation length ‡			0.017 *
<3	35	21 (60.0%)	
≥3	26	6 (23.1%)	
Screw density			0.027 *
<0.67	24	14 (66.7%)	
≥0.67	37	13 (32.5%)	
Fixation method			0.074
Open	46	18 (39.1%)	
Percutaneous	15	9 (60.0%)	

IRC, instrumentation-related complication; SINS, spinal instability neoplastic score; ECOG, Eastern Cooperative Oncology Group; LIV, lowest instrumented vertebra. * Indicates statistical significance (p-value less than 0.05). † SINS 0–6 represents stable, 7–12 potential unstable, and 13–18 unstable. ‡ number of instrumented vertebrae without metastases.

History of radiotherapy, fixation length, and screw density were significantly associated with IRCs ($p = 0.042$, $p = 0.017$, and $p = 0.027$, respectively). Other variables, such as sex, age, primary tumor type, ECOG performance status, BMI, and fixation method showed no significant association with IRCs. A multivariate analysis using Cox proportional-hazards regression was carried out, involving the variables found to be statistically significant during the univariate analysis, and it revealed that only the fixation length was a significant risk factor for IRCs (hazard ratio: 0.358, 95% CI: 0.144–0.888; $p = 0.027$). The median IRC-free survival was 38.1 months (range: 1.0–102.6 months) (Figure 2).

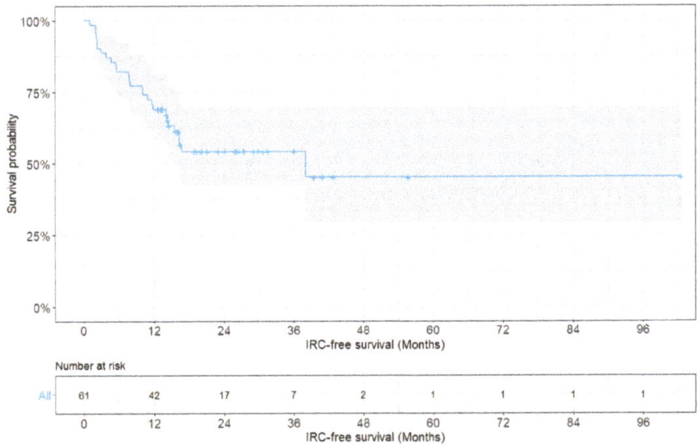

Figure 2. Kaplan–Meier survivorship curve showing instrumentation-related complication-free survival probability for all patients (n = 61).

There was a significant difference in the median IRC-free survival according to the fixation length (15.6 months for a fixation length of less than three vertebrae vs. not reached for a fixation length of three or more vertebrae; $p = 0.017$, log-rank test) (Figure 3).

There was a significant difference in the incidence of IRCs according to the fixation length when the location of the LIV was at or above T10 (8.3% for fixation length < 3 vs. 63.6% for fixation length ≥ 3, $p = 0.007$) (Table 3).

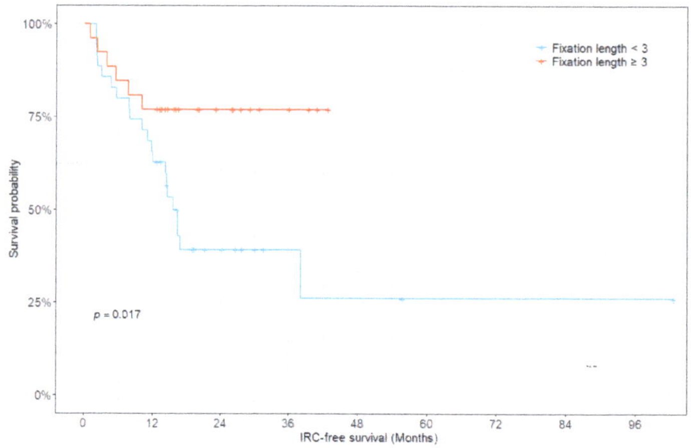

Figure 3. Kaplan–Meier survivorship curve showing instrumentation-related complication-free survival fraction according to the fixation length.

Table 3. Incidence of IRCs with combination of fixation length† and location of the LIV.

	Location of the LIV		p-Value
	At or Above T10	Below T10	
Fixation length † <3	7/11 (63.6%)	14/24 (58.3%)	0.770
Fixation length † ≥3	1/12 (8.3%)	5/14 (35.7%)	0.005 *
p-value	0.007 *	0.105	

IRC, instrumentation-related complication; LIV, lowest instrumented vertebra. * Indicates statistical significance (p-value less than 0.0083) by Mann–Whitney U test. † number of instrumented vertebrae without metastases.

3.1. Illustriative Cases

3.1.1. Case 1

The first patient was a 58-year-old man who was diagnosed with T7 metastasis associated with non–small-cell lung cancer (Figure 4). The T7 metastasis resulted in mechanical back pain. The patient underwent T7 laminectomy and fixation from T6 to T8. Postoperatively, his back pain improved. However, at approximately 12 months after surgery, screw loosening occurred without pain aggravation. At the last follow-up visit (5.8 years after surgery), the patient reported experiencing no significant back pain.

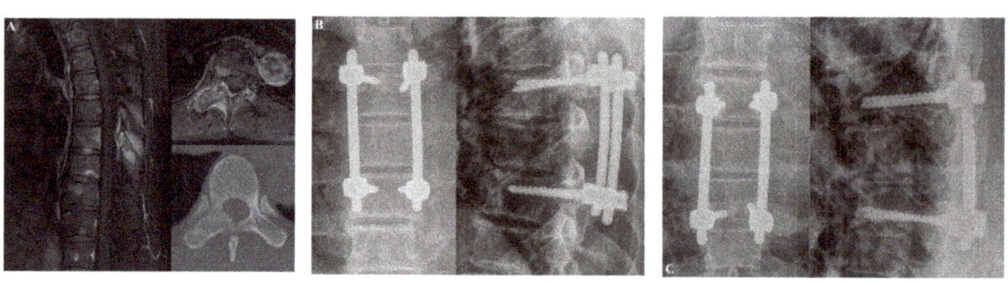

Figure 4. Illustrative case 1. A 58-year-old man was diagnosed with non-small-cell lung cancer metastasis to T7. The patient suffered from mechanical back pain. (**A**) Preoperative T1-weighted enhanced magnetic resonance imaging (MRI) and axial CT scans revealed T7 metastasis. (**B**) At three months after laminectomy with posterior fixation at T6 to T8, his back pain had improved. (**C**) Screw loosening occurred without pain aggravation approximately 12 months after the operation.

3.1.2. Case 2

The second patient was a 60-year-old man who was diagnosed with T12 metastasis associated with non–small-cell lung cancer (Figure 5). The patient had a history of palliative radiotherapy for thoracolumbar spinal metastases (two months prior). The spinal metastasis resulted in right buttock pain that did not subside after the palliative radiotherapy. After laminectomy and fixation from T10 to L2, the buttock pain improved and the patient could walk for an hour. There was no evidence of IRCs at the last follow-up visit (1.5 years after surgery).

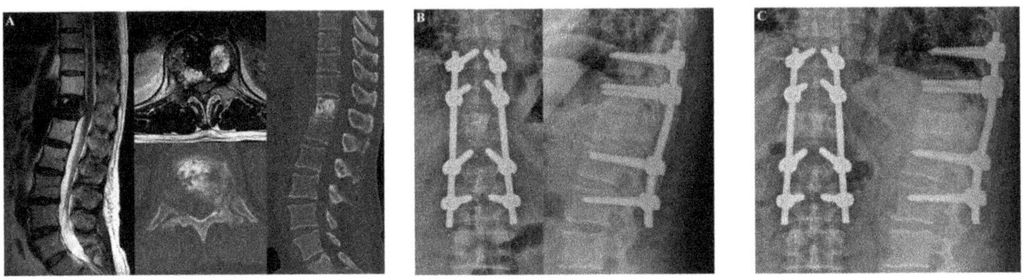

Figure 5. Illustrative case 2. A 60-year-old man was diagnosed with non–small-cell lung cancer metastasis to T12. The patient suffered from buttock pain. (**A**) Preoperative T2-weighted MRI and CT scans revealed T12 metastasis. (**B**) At two weeks after laminectomy with posterior fixation from T10 to L2, the buttock pain improved. (**C**) At the last follow-up, 18 months after the operation, there was no evidence of instrumentation-related complications.

4. Discussion

Obtaining solid bony fusion following instrumentation is considered essential for nononcologic patients to achieve increased construct longevity and better outcomes [5,14]. When spinal fusion is not performed after spinal instrumentation, the risk of developing IRCs increases [15,16]. IRCs, including screw loosening, screw pull-out, and metal breakage, are associated with fatigue on the instrumentation [17]. After spinal fixation, the micromotion within fixed segments exerts repetitive loading on instrumentation [18]. If the fusion procedure is not performed or if solid fusion is not obtained after the fusion procedure, the fatigue applied to the instrumentation accumulates over time and the risk of IRCs increases. Mohi et al. reported that most cases of instrumentation failure occurred before obtaining solid bony fusion [17]. However, fusion procedures can be difficult to perform, and solid bony fusion can be difficult to obtain after the fusion procedure in many patients with MSTs [7]. A longer operation time is necessary, with more bleeding associated with the decortication procedure, and greater costs are associated with the fusion materials [18,19]. Therefore, there is controversy as to whether fusion should be performed in patients with MSTs [8]. Recent studies have reported that satisfactory results after fixation-only surgery can be achieved [7–9,20].

The survival of patients with MSTs varies according to several factors including primary tumor, performance status, and the number of visceral metastases [21]. Chang et al. observed that patients with MSTs survived more than three years after spinal metastases were diagnosed [22]. Shehadi et al. reported that the median survival after the first surgery in patients with MSTs from breast cancer, who are known to have good prognoses, was 21 months (95% CI: 16–27 months) [23]. As systemic treatment has developed, the survival of patients with MSTs has lengthened [1,24], and further studies are required to evaluate whether nonfusion fixation surgery can provoke longevity in patients with MSTs. To evaluate the usefulness of nonfusion surgery as an alternative to fusion surgery, a follow-up period of at least one year, which is longer than the period necessary to achieve solid fusion [25], is required.

In the current study, IRCs occurred in 27 of 61 patients (44.1%) during the mean follow-up period of 28.3 months. Among these, screw loosening was the most common (n = 22 cases). Previous studies have reported that patients with spinal metastases tend to have higher rates of IRCs compared to those with degenerative spinal disorders. This increased risk is believed to be attributable to poor bone quality, systemic disease burden, and the effects of adjuvant therapies such as radiotherapy and chemotherapy. While the reported incidence of IRCs in degenerative spine disease ranges from 0.85% to 10.4% [26,27], studies in metastatic spine tumor patients have shown a higher incidence, typically ranging from 10% to 40% [8,28]. Our findings are consistent with this trend, demonstrating a relatively high frequency of IRCs in this patient population. When comparing the incidence of IRCs between the early (2005–2012) and late (2013–2018) periods, no significant difference was observed (46.2% vs. 43.8%). In a previous study, we reported nine cases (6.4%) of IRCs in 140 operations and three cases (2.2%) of symptomatic IRCs in 136 patients during a mean follow-up period of 16.5 months [9]. Drakhshandeh et al. reported zero cases of IRCs in 27 patients during a mean follow-up period of 12.2 months [8]. There were reasons for why the incidence of IRCs in the present study was much higher than that in previous studies. First, our present study had a longer mean follow-up period relative to those of other studies. Second, the definition of IRCs varied. Drakhshandeh et al.'s study did not include screw loosening in the definition of IRCs. In the current study, the number IRCs excluding screw loosening totaled five cases (8.1%), which is not significantly different from those reported in previous studies. Of the 61 patients in the current study, three (4.9%) experienced pain related to IRCs at a mean of 4.3 months after surgery, although only one patient (1.6%) underwent intervention via cement augmentation. Despite the majority of the IRCs being asymptomatic, initial instrumentation was considered necessary to achieve spinal stability and prevent neurologic deterioration in this vulnerable patient population. Amankulor et al. reported nine cases of symptomatic IRCs in 318 patients and a median of 39.9 months of IRC-free survival [28]. Even though the follow-up period of our study was longer than that of other studies, it was not significantly different when compared to previous studies. The median IRC-free survival period was 38.1 months, whereas the median overall survival period was 35.6 months. Even the median overall survival period after surgery in our study was longer than in previous studies [22,23], while the median IRC-free survival length exceeded the median overall survival length. This suggests the longevity of fixation surgery without fusion in patients with MST.

In our study, the primary risk factor for IRCs was fixation length, which was defined as the number of instrumented vertebrae without metastases, because the number of vertebrae with metastases also affected the construct length. When one-above and one-below pedicle screw fixation over vertebrae with metastases was performed, the fixation length was two. A fixation length of three or more vertebrae significantly decreased the risk of IRCs. The long fixation length increased the stability in the spinal column, while the short fixation length increased the construct failure and loss of correction [29]. Amankulor et al. reported that construct length was one of the risk factors for IRC onset after surgery in patients with MSTs [28].

Although adopting a long fixation length reduces the risk of IRCs, it has several disadvantages. For example, it loses more motion segments, affects adjacent segments with larger bending moments, and necessitates more operation time to complete. Since the thoracic spine has more stiffness than the lumbar spine because of the presence of the rib cage [30], the adequate fixation length will vary depending on the location of the construct. In the current study, if the fixation length was three or more vertebrae, the incidence of

IRCs was decreased relative to when the fixation length was less than three vertebrae, regardless of the location of the LIV. However, when the fixation length was three or more vertebrae, the incidence of IRCs was significantly smaller when the LIV was located at or above T10. The incidence of IRCs might be decreased in the thoracic region because the thoracic spine achieves less bending movements due to the presence of the rib cage. McLain et al. reported that the involvement of a long fixation construct has an advantage in the thoracic area, whereas shorter fixation constructs have an advantage in the lumbar area [31].

Several limitations should be acknowledged. The small sample size and retrospective design limit the statistical power of the study and introduce a potential risk of information bias. Additionally, this study may have overestimated the overall survival and IRC-free survival, as patients with less than one year of follow-up were excluded. This exclusion was intentional, as our primary aim was to assess the long-term mechanical durability of nonfusion constructs. Early postoperative complications may be affected by systemic factors such as disease progression or surgical complexity rather than construct mechanics. Including patients who died early may have introduced confounding factors unrelated to implant performance. The radiographic evaluations were not standardized, with both plain radiographs and CT scans used. Notably, the IRCs may have been underestimated because CT imaging is less sensitive than plain radiography for detecting screw loosening [32]. Although bone mineral density (BMD) was not routinely measured in the included patients and therefore not analyzed, it may influence the risk of instrumentation-related complications. We acknowledge the absence of BMD data as a limitation. Likewise, systemic treatments such as bisphosphonates, immunotherapy, or targeted therapy were not specifically considered in the analysis. Although these therapies can potentially affect bone healing and implant stability, detailed treatment data were not uniformly available in the medical records. We acknowledge this as another limitation of our study. Furthermore, cement augmentation, or kyphoplasty, was not performed in any of the included cases. Considering the relatively high incidence of IRCs such as screw loosening, these adjunctive procedures may have provided additional construct stability. Their potential role should be explored in future studies, particularly in patients with compromised bone quality. Likewise, spinal alignment was not independently analyzed as a variable; however, it may have been indirectly accounted for through the SINS criteria, which include components related to deformity. Implant size, particularly screw diameter, was not statistically assessed, although the largest possible pedicle screws were used intraoperatively based on surgeon judgment. Furthermore, this study focused solely on radiographic outcomes and did not include data on clinical outcomes. Finally, because patients who underwent fusion with instrumentation were not included, a direct comparison between nonfusion and fusion surgery was not possible.

Given that the mean IRC-free survival was 9.6 months and that most of the IRCs occurred within the first postoperative year, we recommend routine radiographic surveillance at 3, 6, and 12 months postoperatively, followed by annual imaging. If IRC is identified at 6 months or if symptoms are present, interim imaging at 9 months may be beneficial to monitor progression or symptom correlation.

5. Conclusions

The current study reported that IRCs were frequent but mostly asymptomatic following posterior fixation without fusion in patients with MSTs followed up for at least one year. The IRC-free survival was long enough considering the actual survival of patient. Longer fixation lengths of three or more vertebrae reduced IRCs regardless of the MST location, but the IRCs were more significantly reduced when the location of the LIV was at or above T10.

Author Contributions: Conceptualization, S.-J.P. and C.-S.L.; methodology, Y.N. and S.-J.P.; validation, Y.N., J.-S.P. and D.-H.K.; formal analysis, Y.N. and S.-J.P.; resources, S.-J.P. and C.-S.L.; data curation, Y.N.; writing—original draft preparation, Y.N.; writing—review and editing, S.-J.P.; visualization, J.-S.P. and D.-H.K.; supervision, S.-J.P., C.-S.L. and S.W.S.; project administration, S.-J.P. and C.-S.L. All authors have read and agreed to the published version of the manuscript.

Funding: This research received no external funding.

Institutional Review Board Statement: This study was conducted in accordance with the Declaration of Helsinki, and approved by the Institutional Review Board of Samsung Medical Center (IRB number: 2020-08-138-001, 3 September 2020).

Informed Consent Statement: Patient consent was waived due to the retrospective nature of this study.

Data Availability Statement: The data underlying this article cannot be shared publicly because of the privacy of the individuals who participated in this study. The data can be shared by the corresponding author upon reasonable request.

Conflicts of Interest: The authors declare no conflicts of interest. The funders had no role in the design of the study; in the collection, analyses, or interpretation of data; in the writing of the manuscript; or in the decision to publish the results.

References

1. Murotani, K.; Fujibayashi, S.; Otsuki, B.; Shimizu, T.; Sono, T.; Onishi, E.; Kimura, H.; Tamaki, Y.; Tsubouchi, N.; Ota, M. Prognostic factors after surgical treatment for spinal metastases. *Asian Spine J.* **2024**, *18*, 390. [CrossRef] [PubMed]
2. Sugita, S.; Hozumi, T.; Yamakawa, K.; Goto, T. The significance of spinal fixation in palliative surgery for spinal metastases. *J. Clin. Neurosci.* **2018**, *48*, 163–167. [CrossRef] [PubMed]
3. Falicov, A.; Fisher, C.G.; Sparkes, J.; Boyd, M.C.; Wing, P.C.; Dvorak, M.F. Impact of surgical intervention on quality of life in patients with spinal metastases. *Spine* **2006**, *31*, 2849–2856. [CrossRef] [PubMed]
4. Tang, Y.; Qu, J.; Wu, J.; Liu, H.; Chu, T.; Xiao, J.; Zhou, Y. Effect of Surgery on Quality of Life of Patients with Spinal Metastasis from Non-Small-Cell Lung Cancer. *J. Bone Jt. Surg. Am.* **2016**, *98*, 396–402. [CrossRef]
5. Vrionis, F.D.; Small, J. Surgical management of metastatic spinal neoplasms. *Neurosurg. Focus.* **2003**, *15*, 1–8. [CrossRef]
6. Tian, N.F.; Wu, Y.S.; Zhang, X.L.; Wu, X.L.; Chi, Y.L.; Mao, F.M. Fusion versus nonfusion for surgically treated thoracolumbar burst fractures: A meta-analysis. *PLoS ONE* **2013**, *8*, e63995. [CrossRef]
7. Bellato, R.T.; Teixeira, W.G.; Torelli, A.G.; Cristante, A.F.; de Barros, T.E.; de Camargo, O.P. Late failure of posterior fixation without bone fusion for vertebral metastases. *Acta Ortop. Bras.* **2015**, *23*, 303–306. [CrossRef]
8. Drakhshandeh, D.; Miller, J.A.; Fabiano, A.J. Instrumented Spinal Stabilization without Fusion for Spinal Metastatic Disease. *World Neurosurg.* **2018**, *111*, e403–e409. [CrossRef]
9. Park, S.J.; Lee, K.H.; Lee, C.S.; Jung, J.Y.; Park, J.H.; Kim, G.L.; Kim, K.T. Instrumented surgical treatment for metastatic spinal tumors: Is fusion necessary? *J. Neurosurg. Spine* **2019**, 1–9. [CrossRef]
10. Sanden, B.; Olerud, C.; Petren-Mallmin, M.; Johansson, C.; Larsson, S. The significance of radiolucent zones surrounding pedicle screws. Definition of screw loosening in spinal instrumentation. *J. Bone Jt. Surg. Br.* **2004**, *86*, 457–461. [CrossRef]
11. Fisher, C.G.; DiPaola, C.P.; Ryken, T.C.; Bilsky, M.H.; Shaffrey, C.I.; Berven, S.H.; Harrop, J.S.; Fehlings, M.G.; Boriani, S.; Chou, D. A novel classification system for spinal instability in neoplastic disease: An evidence-based approach and expert consensus from the Spine Oncology Study Group. *Spine* **2010**, *35*, E1221–E1229. [CrossRef] [PubMed]
12. Newman, W.C.; Amin, A.G.; Villavieja, J.; Laufer, I.; Bilsky, M.H.; Barzilai, O. Short-segment cement-augmented fixation in open separation surgery of metastatic epidural spinal cord compression: Initial experience. *Neurosurg. Focus.* **2021**, *50*, E11. [CrossRef] [PubMed]
13. Clements, D.H.; Betz, R.R.; Newton, P.O.; Rohmiller, M.; Marks, M.C.; Bastrom, T. Correlation of scoliosis curve correction with the number and type of fixation anchors. *Spine* **2009**, *34*, 2147–2150. [CrossRef] [PubMed]
14. Kim, Y.-H.; Kim, K.-W.; Rhyu, K.-W.; Park, J.-B.; Shin, J.-H.; Kim, Y.-Y.; Lee, J.-S.; Ahn, J.-H.; Ryu, J.-H.; Park, H.-Y. Bone fusion materials: Past, present, and future. *Asian Spine J.* **2025**, *19*, 490–500. [CrossRef]

15. Wetzel, F.T.; Brustein, M.; Phillips, F.M.; Trott, S. Hardware failure in an unconstrained lumbar pedicle screw system: A 2-year follow-up study. *Spine* **1999**, *24*, 1138–1143. [CrossRef]
16. Jutte, P.C.; Castelein, R.M. Complications of pedicle screws in lumbar and lumbosacral fusions in 105 consecutive primary operations. *Eur. Spine J.* **2002**, *11*, 594–598. [CrossRef]
17. Mohi Eldin, M.M.; Ali, A.M.A. Lumbar Transpedicular Implant Failure: A Clinical and Surgical Challenge and Its Radiological Assessment. *Asian Spine J.* **2014**, *8*, 281. [CrossRef]
18. Ferrara, L.A.; Secor, J.L.; Jin, B.-h.; Wakefield, A.; Inceoglu, S.; Benzel, E.C. A biomechanical comparison of facet screw fixation and pedicle screw fixation: Effects of short-term and long-term repetitive cycling. *Spine* **2003**, *28*, 1226–1234. [CrossRef]
19. Glassman, S.D.; Carreon, L.Y.; Campbell, M.J.; Johnson, J.R.; Puno, R.M.; Djurasovic, M.; Dimar, J.R. The perioperative cost of Infuse bone graft in posterolateral lumbar spine fusion. *Spine J.* **2008**, *8*, 443–448. [CrossRef]
20. Pedreira, R.; Abu-Bonsrah, N.; Karim Ahmed, A.; De la Garza-Ramos, R.; Rory Goodwin, C.; Gokaslan, Z.L.; Sacks, J.; Sciubba, D.M. Hardware failure in patients with metastatic cancer to the spine. *J. Clin. Neurosci.* **2017**, *45*, 166–171. [CrossRef]
21. Switlyk, M.D.; Kongsgaard, U.; Skjeldal, S.; Hald, J.K.; Hole, K.H.; Knutstad, K.; Zaikova, O. Prognostic factors in patients with symptomatic spinal metastases and normal neurological function. *Clin. Oncol.* **2015**, *27*, 213–221. [CrossRef] [PubMed]
22. Chang, S.Y.; Ha, J.H.; Seo, S.G.; Chang, B.S.; Lee, C.K.; Kim, H. Prognosis of Single Spinal Metastatic Tumors: Predictive Value of the Spinal Instability Neoplastic Score System for Spinal Adverse Events. *Asian Spine J.* **2018**, *12*, 919–926. [CrossRef] [PubMed]
23. Shehadi, J.A.; Sciubba, D.M.; Suk, I.; Suki, D.; Maldaun, M.V.; McCutcheon, I.E.; Nader, R.; Theriault, R.; Rhines, L.D.; Gokaslan, Z.L. Surgical treatment strategies and outcome in patients with breast cancer metastatic to the spine: A review of 87 patients. *Eur. Spine J.* **2007**, *16*, 1179–1192. [CrossRef] [PubMed]
24. Wright, E.; Ricciardi, F.; Arts, M.; Buchowski, J.M.; Chung, C.K.; Coppes, M.; Crockard, A.; Depreitere, B.; Fehlings, M.; Kawahara, N.; et al. Metastatic Spine Tumor Epidemiology: Comparison of Trends in Surgery Across Two Decades and Three Continents. *World Neurosurg.* **2018**, *114*, e809–e817. [CrossRef]
25. Ravindra, V.M.; Godzik, J.; Dailey, A.T.; Schmidt, M.H.; Bisson, E.F.; Hood, R.S.; Cutler, A.; Ray, W.Z. Vitamin D Levels and 1-Year Fusion Outcomes in Elective Spine Surgery: A Prospective Observational Study. *Spine* **2015**, *40*, 1536–1541. [CrossRef]
26. Shillingford, J.N.; Laratta, J.L.; Sarpong, N.O.; Alrabaa, R.G.; Cerpa, M.K.; Lehman, R.A.; Lenke, L.G.; Fischer, C.R. Instrumentation complication rates following spine surgery: A report from the Scoliosis Research Society (SRS) morbidity and mortality database. *J. Spine Surg.* **2019**, *5*, 110. [CrossRef]
27. Demura, S.; Ohara, T.; Tauchi, R.; Takimura, K.; Watanabe, K.; Suzuki, S.; Uno, K.; Suzuki, T.; Yanagida, H.; Yamaguchi, T. Incidence and causes of instrument-related complications after primary definitive fusion for pediatric spine deformity. *J. Neurosurg. Spine* **2022**, *38*, 192–198. [CrossRef]
28. Amankulor, N.M.; Xu, R.; Iorgulescu, J.B.; Chapman, T.; Reiner, A.S.; Riedel, E.; Lis, E.; Yamada, Y.; Bilsky, M.; Laufer, I. The incidence and patterns of hardware failure after separation surgery in patients with spinal metastatic tumors. *Spine J.* **2014**, *14*, 1850–1859. [CrossRef]
29. Mikles, M.R.; Stchur, R.P.; Graziano, G.P. Posterior instrumentation for thoracolumbar fractures. *JAAOS-J. Am. Acad. Orthop. Surg.* **2004**, *12*, 424–435. [CrossRef]
30. Mannen, E.M.; Friis, E.A.; Sis, H.L.; Wong, B.M.; Cadel, E.S.; Anderson, D.E. The rib cage stiffens the thoracic spine in a cadaveric model with body weight load under dynamic moments. *J. Mech. Behav. Biomed. Mater.* **2018**, *84*, 258–264. [CrossRef]
31. McLain, R.F. The biomechanics of long versus short fixation for thoracolumbar spine fractures. *Spine* **2006**, *31*, S70–S79. [CrossRef]
32. Galbusera, F.; Volkheimer, D.; Reitmaier, S.; Berger-Roscher, N.; Kienle, A.; Wilke, H.J. Pedicle screw loosening: A clinically relevant complication? *Eur. Spine J.* **2015**, *24*, 1005–1016. [CrossRef]

Journal of
Clinical Medicine

MDPI

Article

BioGlue® Induced Mass Formation Aggravating Spinal Canal Invasion After Intradural Tumor Surgery

Sun Woo Jang [1], Sang Hyub Lee [2], Hong Kyung Shin [3], Sang Ryong Jeon [3], Danbi Park [3,4], Chongman Kim [5] and Jin Hoon Park [3,*]

1 Department of Neurological Surgery, Gangneung Asan Hospital, University of Ulsan College of Medicine, Gangneung 25440, Republic of Korea; sunwoo0118@naver.com
2 Department of Neurosurgery, Spine Center, The Leon Wiltse Memorial Hospital, Suwon 16499, Republic of Korea; shlee.kns@gmail.com
3 Department of Neurological Surgery, Asan Medical Center, University of Ulsan College of Medicine, Seoul 05505, Republic of Korea; mxshin@gmail.com (H.K.S.); srjeon190@gmail.com (S.R.J.); danbi08@kakao.com (D.P.)
4 College of Nursing, Korea University, Seoul 02841, Republic of Korea
5 Department of Industrial and Management Engineering, Myongji University, Seoul 03674, Republic of Korea; chongman@mju.ac.kr
* Correspondence: spinejhpark@naver.com; Tel.: +82-2-3010-3550

Abstract: Background/Objectives: The aim of this study was to evaluate whether the use of BioGlue® increases the risk of postoperative mass formation and subsequent spinal canal invasion after intradural spinal tumor surgery. **Methods**: After retrospectively reviewing patients who underwent intradural tumor surgery from 2018 to 2023, we evaluated mass formation as detected in postoperative MRI according to the Epidural Spinal Cord Compression (ESCC) grade. Patients were divided into two groups based on the use of BioGlue®, and we analyzed MRI postoperatively to compare the differences in ESCC grades and the incidence of symptomatic spinal canal invasion between the two groups. Additionally, we performed a logistic regression analysis to identify risk factors associated with mass formation and to explore their relationship with BioGlue®. **Results**: This study included a total of 153 patients, 87 in the BioGlue® and 66 in the non-BioGlue® groups. In the BioGlue® group, 18 patients had ESCC grade 2, and 11 had grade 3. Conversely, in the non-BioGlue® group, only 8 patients had ESCC grade 2, and none had grade 3 ($p = 0.001$). Among the cases of symptomatic spinal canal invasion, all five cases were identified in the BioGlue® group ($p = 0.001$). Both univariate and multivariate analyses showed that BioGlue® was a significant risk factor for spinal canal invasion (univariate: OR = 3.931, $p = 0.005$, multivariate: OR = 3.812, $p = 0.003$). **Conclusions**: Our findings indicated that BioGlue® was a significant risk factor for mass formation aggravating spinal canal invasion after intradural tumor surgery.

Keywords: cerebrospinal fluid leak; intradural spinal cord tumor; spinal canal invasion; BioGlue®

1. Introduction

BioGlue® (CryoLife, Atlanta, GA, USA) is a surgical sealant consisting of bovine serum albumin and glutaraldehyde (BSAG) that polymerizes within 20 to 30 s when mixed. A common adjunct to achieve hemostasis during the surgical repair of large vessels such as the aorta, femoral, and carotid arteries [1,2], BioGlue® is also frequently used in off-label applications in neurosurgery to prevent cerebrospinal fluid (CSF) leakage.

This has been supported by several reports discussing its effectiveness in CSF leakage repair [3–6]. However, the product has yet to receive official, full approval for such use [3,7,8], mainly due to concerns about mass effects, neurotoxicity, and infection [9–11]. Reports in the Manufacturer and User Facility Device Experience (MAUDE) databases have routinely documented mass effects associated with BioGlue® used in dural repairs. While a few case reports exist on the side effects of BioGlue® as a dural sealant [5,12,13], a more comprehensive, systematic study is yet to be published. Moreover, in South Korea, BioGlue® is covered by insurance to prevent CSF leakage in neurosurgical procedures. Thus, we aimed to assess the potential risks associated with the use of BioGlue®, particularly its relationship with spinal canal invasion and neurological deterioration. We compared radiologic and surgical outcomes between BioGlue® and non-BioGlue® groups to identify its adverse effects in spine surgery.

2. Materials and Methods

This study was approved by the Institutional Review Board (IRB, No. 2023-1613), ensuring compliance with ethical standards. Given the retrospective nature of the study, the IRB waived the requirement for informed consent.

2.1. Study Design and Participants

We retrospectively reviewed 250 patients who received intradural spinal cord tumor removal surgery from March 2018 to January 2023 and selected 153 after excluding those with any of the following: (1) epidural spinal cord tumor surgery without durotomy, (2) revision surgery, (3) procedure other than laminoplastic laminotomy, and (4) no postoperative MRI or insufficient medical record.

2.2. Surgical Procedures

We performed laminoplastic laminotomy at the surgical level on the spinal cord tumor (Figure 1A) and midline durotomy to expose the spinal cord tumor (Figure 1B). After removing the spinal cord tumor, we closed the dura using Prolene 5-0 and 6-0 sutures (Figure 1C), and the lateral side dura defect from the inside in the same manner after removing a dumbbell-shaped schwannoma. Moreover, we selectively applied adjunctive materials such as a collagen patch (TachoComb®; Baxter, Inc., Deerfield, IL, USA) or non-soluble glue (BioGlue®) based on the surgeon's decision. In cases, we selectively used either BioGlue® or TachoComb®. However, in instances of durotomy involving more than two levels or a weak dura, we employed both products (Figure 1D). To avoid postoperative mass effects, we applied a 1 mm-thin layer of BioGlue® to the epidural space as recommended in a previous study [14] (Figure 1E). Finally, we performed the Valsalva maneuver to screen for unresolved CSF leakage and laminoplasty, followed by layer-by-layer muscle and skin closure using Vicryl and nylon.

2.3. Postoperative Follow-Up

In the postoperative state, patients were encouraged to start ambulation on the day after surgery. A follow-up MRI was performed within one week postoperatively to screen for any abnormal findings, such as residual tumor or CSF leakage. If nothing specific was detected on the postoperative MRI and signs of infection or wound dehiscence were not found, the patients were discharged and asked to revisit the outpatient clinic in a month. After confirming the pathology, the follow-up plan for the patients was established. If confirmed as a benign tumor, a follow-up MRI was planned three years after surgery. If diagnosed as a malignant tumor, short-term follow-up with adjuvant therapy such as radiotherapy or chemotherapy was scheduled. During the follow-up period, revision surgery was performed if postoperative complications such as CSF leakage, wound infection, or neurologic deterioration—such as motor weakness due to a mass formation invading the spinal canal found in follow-up MRI—occurred.

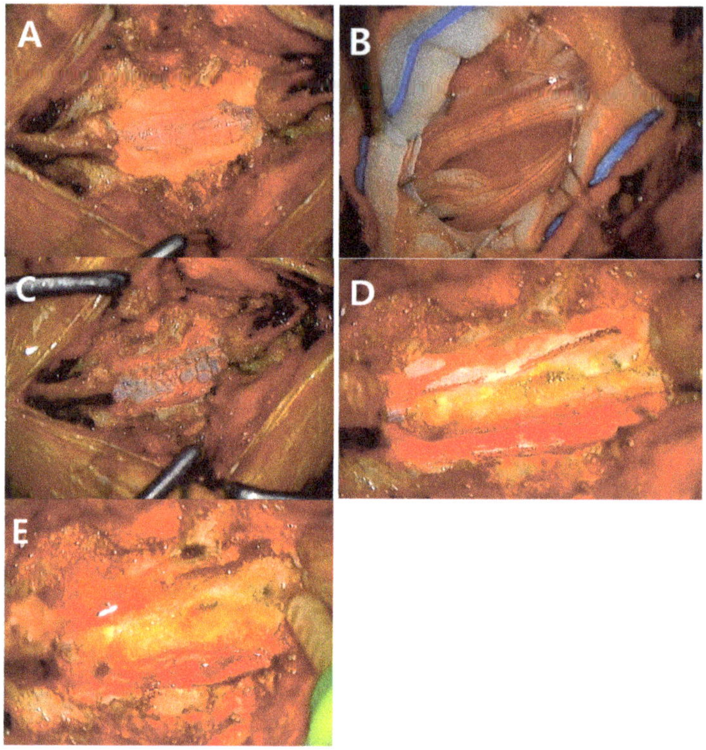

Figure 1. Surgical procedure for spinal cord tumor surgery. Surgical laminectomy or laminoplastic laminotomy was performed at the spinal cord tumor (**A**), and midline durotomy was performed to expose the spinal cord tumor (**B**). After spinal cord tumor resection, dura was closed using Prolene 5-0 and 6-0 sutures (**C**), and adjunctive materials such as a collagen patch (TachoComb®; Baxter, Inc., IL, USA) or non-soluble glue (BioGlue®) were applied selectively (**D**). A 1 mm-thin layer of BioGlue® was applied to the epidural space as recommended in a previous study to avoid any post-operative mass effect [14] (**E**). Then, laminoplasty was performed depending on the surgical plan, followed by layer-by-layer muscle and skin closure using Vicryl and nylon.

2.4. Radiological Analysis

By examining the postoperative MRI of the 153 enrolled patients, we revealed that spinal canal invading lesions appeared as a low signal on T2 images. While the epidural lesions could initially be considered as hematomas in the postoperative state, hematomas were isodense on T2 MR images, gradually becoming hypointense and then hyperintense after one week in the hyperacute stage [15,16]. On the other hand, epidural compressing lesions found as hypointense on T2 MR images in this study remained in a follow-up MRI conducted a few months after surgery, suggesting they were not simple hematomas. Additionally, BioGlue® is known to manifest a low signal in T2 MR images [17,18]. Hence, it was assumed that a mass displaying low signal intensity in a T2 MR image was directly correlated with the effects of BioGlue®.

The postoperative MRI results were classified based on the Epidural Spinal Cord Compression (ESCC) grading system, originally designed to differentiate the extent of cord compression in metastatic spine tumors to guide surgical intervention [19]: grade 1 with epidural extension without cord compression; grade 2 with spinal cord compression and visible CSF around the spinal cord; and grade 3 with spinal cord compression and no visible CSF near the spinal cord. The patients were categorized into the BioGlue® and the non-BioGlue® groups, depending on the post-dural suture use of BioGlue®, to compare the incidences of ESCC grades.

2.5. Postoperative Complication Analysis

Postoperative complications requiring revision surgery were collected and classified into the BioGlue® and non-BioGlue® groups to analyze the relationship between the incidence of revision surgery and the use of BioGlue®.

2.6. Analysis of ESCC Grades 2 and 3 Risk Factors

To diversify our perspectives, we also analyzed numerous risk factors for spinal canal invasion with ESCC grades 2 and 3, including age, sex, type of operation, surgical location, surgical level, and the use of BioGlue® or Tachocomb®, as well as the relationship between these factors and ESCC grades 2 and 3.

2.7. Statistical Analysis

Simple t-tests to compare the BioGlue® and non-BioGlue® groups were conducted using SPSS version 20.0 (IBM, Chicago, IL, USA), with statistical significance set at $p < 0.05$. Logistic regression was conducted to generate estimates of odds ratios (OR) and 95% confidence intervals (CIs) to examine the relationship between the investigated risk factors and ESCC grades 2 and 3.

3. Results

3.1. Demographics

Table 1 presents the demographic data of the enrolled patients categorized into three groups stratified by ESCC grade. The ESCC grade 1 group had 116 patients, with 51 men (43.9%) and a mean age of 52.8 ± 16.4. The ESCC grade 2 group had 26 patients, with six men (23.1%) and a mean age of 53.2 ± 16.6. The ESCC grade 3 group had 11 patients, including five men (45.4%) and a mean age of 52.9 ± 16.4. Among the 116 ESCC grade 1 patients, 25 (21.5%) were diagnosed with meningioma, 63 (54.4%) with schwannoma, and 13 (11.2%) with ependymoma. Among the 26 ESCC grade 2 patients, 8 (30.7%) were diagnosed with meningioma, 10 (38.4%) with schwannoma, and 6 (23.1%) with ependymoma. Among the 11 ESCC grade 3 patients, 3 (27.3%) were diagnosed with meningioma, 4 (36.3%) with schwannoma, and none (0%) with ependymoma. The three groups showed no statistically significant difference in tumor type ($p = 0.272$).

Next, 29 (25%) patients had a cervical level, 49 (42.2%) a thoracic level, and 38 (32.8%) a lumbosacral level spinal cord tumor in the ESCC grade 1 group; 13 (50%) patients had a cervical level, 10 (38.4%) a thoracic level, and 3 (11.6%) a lumbosacral level spinal cord tumor in the ESCC grade 2 group; and 5 (45.4%) patients had a cervical level, 4 (36.3%) a thoracic level, and 2 (18.3%) a lumbosacral level spinal cord tumor in the ESCC grade 3 group, proving no statistically significant difference between the three groups ($p = 0.141$).

A total of 26 (22.4%) patients had one level surgery, 71 (61.2%) two levels, and 19 (16.4%) three levels or more in the ESCC grade 1 group; 1 (3.9%) patient had one level surgery, 13 (50%) two levels, and 12 (46.1%) had three levels or more in the ESCC grade 2 group; and 3 (27.3%) patients had one level surgery, 5 (45.4%) two levels, and 3 (27.3%) had three levels or more in the ESCC grade 3 group, also confirming no statistically significant difference between the three groups ($p = 0.761$).

Table 1. Demographics of patients who underwent intradural tumor surgery stratified by ESCC Grade.

	ESCC Grade			p-Value
	Grade 1 (n = 116)	Grade 2 (n = 26)	Grade 3 (n = 11)	
Age (yrs)	52.8 ± 16.4	53.2 ± 16.6	52.9 ± 16.4	0.392
Sex				0.923
male	51 (43.9)	6 (23.1)	5 (45.4)	
Pathology				0.272
Meningioma	25 (21.5)	8 (30.7)	3 (27.3)	
Schwannoma	63 (54.4)	10 (38.4)	4 (36.3)	
Neurofibroma	2 (1.7)	0 (0)	1 (9.1)	
Ependymoma	13 (11.2)	6 (23.1)	0 (0)	
Glioma	2 (1.7)	0 (0)	1 (9.1)	
Hemangiobloastoma	3 (2.6)	0 (0)	0 (0)	
Cavernous malformation	2 (1.7)	0 (0)	0 (0)	
Metastasis	3 (2.6)	1 (3.9)	1 (9.1)	
Others	3 (2.6)	1 (3.9)	1 (9.1)	
Tumor location				0.141
Cervical	29 (25)	13 (50)	5 (45.4)	
Thoracic	49 (42.2)	10 (38.4)	4 (36.3)	
Lumbosacral	38 (32.8)	3 (11.6)	2 (18.3)	
Operation level				0.761
1 level	26 (22.4)	1 (3.9)	3 (27.3)	
2 levels	71 (61.2)	13 (50)	5 (45.4)	
≥3 levels	19 (16.4)	12 (46.1)	3 (27.3)	
Use of Bioglue®	58 (50)	18 (69.2)	11 (100)	0.001 ***
Use of TachoComb®	107 (92.2)	24 (92.3)	9 (81.8)	0.240

ESCC grade: epidural spinal cord compression scale; others included chordoma, neuroenteric cyst, hemangioma, benign cyst, granulation, atypical lymphocyte; *** $p < 0.001$.

Finally, 107 (92.2%) patients in ESCC grade 1 groups, 24 (92.3%) in grade 2 groups, and 9 (91.8%) in grade 3 groups used TachoComb®, which revealed no statistically significant difference ($p = 0.240$). However, 58 (50%) patients in the ESCC grade 1 groups, 18 (69.2%) in ESCC grade 2 groups, and 11 (100%) in ESCC grade 3 groups used Bioglue®, which revealed a statistically significant difference between the three groups ($p = 0.001$).

3.2. ESCC Grade Analysis

A comparison of the postoperative MRIs of the BioGlue® and non-BioGlue® groups using the ESCC grade scale demonstrated that 58 patients (66.7%) in the BioGlue® group had grade 1, 18 (20.7%) had grade 2, and 11 (12.6%) had grade 3, while 58 patients (87.9%) in the non-BioGlue® group had grade 1, 8 (12.1%) had grade 2, and no patient had grade 3. This confirmed a statistically notable difference between the two groups (p value = 0.001) (Table 2).

Table 2. ESCC grade and complications in the BioGlue® and non-BioGlue® groups.

	BioGlue® (n = 87)	Non-BioGlue® (n = 66)	p-Value
ESCC Grade			0.001 ***
grade 1	58 (66.7)	58 (87.9)	
grade 2	18 (20.7)	8 (12.1)	
grade 3	11 (12.6)	0 (0.0)	
Symptomatic spinal canal invasion	5 (5.7)	0 (0.0)	0.001 ***
CSF leakage	1 (1.1)	0 (0.0)	0.080

ESCC grade: epidural spinal cord compression scale; CSF: cerebrospinal fluid leakage; *** $p < 0.001$.

3.3. Review of Revision Cases

Out of the 153 enrolled patients, a total of seven cases required revision surgery due to postoperative complications at the surgical site (Table 3). Among them, five cases were correlated with delayed mass formation aggravating spinal canal invasion. A 50-year-old female patient was diagnosed with an intradural spinal cord tumor at the C5-6 level (Figure 2A) and underwent laminoplastic laminotomy at C5-6 with resection of the intradural spinal cord tumor. Postoperative MR revealed no residual tumor (Figure 2B), and pathology confirmed the tumor as a neurofibroma. Two months postoperatively, the patient experienced weakness in all four extremities, and a follow-up MRI confirmed a severe cord compressing lesion (Figure 2C), leading to her readmission for further evaluation. Initially, a laboratory study was conducted under the suspicion of a postoperative abscess, but it found no clinical signs or lab abnormalities suggesting an infection; ultimately, a diagnostic revisional surgery was performed. During the revision surgeries, a mass compressing the spinal cord was identified, accompanied by a yellowish fluid inside with moderate to severe spinal cord adhesions (Figure 2D). However, culture studies of the yellowish fluid in the postoperative state did not detect any specific bacteria or signs of infection (Figure 2E). Furthermore, no white blood cells or epithelial cells were detected in the sample. In four other patients, postoperative neurological deterioration was observed, with mass formation invading into the spinal canal identified in their follow-up MRI, ranging from POD 1 to 8 months, prompting revision surgeries. All five cases belonged to the BioGlue® group.

Table 3. Revision cases due to complications.

No.	Age	Sex	Diagnosis	Operation	BioGlue®	Complication
1	56	M	Schwannoma	LP, L1	Yes	POD 1 mo MRI compression lesion
2	30	F	Schwannoma	LP, L5	Yes	POD 4 mo progressing motor weakness, MRI compression lesion
3	38	F	Meningioma	LP, C3-6	Yes	POD 1 mo progressing motor weakness, MRI compression lesion
4	50	F	Neurofibroma	LP, C5-6	Yes	POD 2 mo progressing motor weakness, MRI compression lesion
5	63	F	Meningioma	LP, C5-7	Yes	POD 8 mo progressing motor weakness, MRI compression lesion
6	80	M	Schwannoma	LP, S1	Yes	CSF leakage
7	76	F	Meningioma	LP, S1	Yes	POD 3 d NOAC restart due to pulmonary embolism, and subsequent postoperative epidural hematoma

LP: Laminoplasty; POD: postoperative date; NOAC: non-vitamin K antagonist oral anticoagulants.

Additionally, one patient in the BioGlue® group had a follow-up MRI confirming operative site bulging and CSF leakage. Another case involved a postoperative pulmonary embolism; non-vitamin K antagonist oral anticoagulants (NOAC) were started on day three after surgery. Neurological deterioration and hematoma were identified on follow-up MRI, necessitating revision surgery.

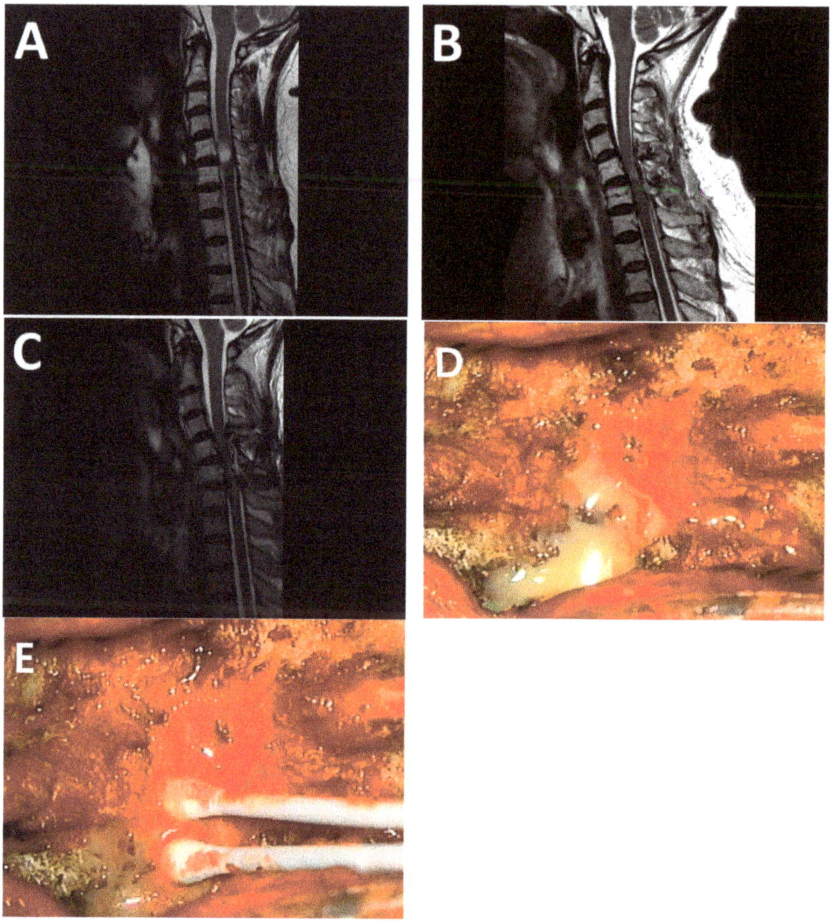

Figure 2. Representative cases of symptomatic cord compression and revision surgery. A 50-year-old female patient was diagnosed with an intradural spinal cord tumor at C5-6 level (**A**) and underwent laminoplastic laminotomy at C5-6 with resection of the intradural spinal cord tumor. Postoperative MR revealed no residual tumor (**B**), and pathology confirmed the tumor as a neurofibroma. Two months postoperatively, the patient experienced weakness in all four extremities, and a follow-up MRI confirmed a severe cord compressing lesion (**C**), leading to her readmission for further evaluation. Initially, a laboratory study was conducted under the suspicion of a postoperative abscess, but it found no clinical signs or lab abnormalities suggesting an infection. Ultimately, diagnostic revisional surgery was performed. During the revision surgeries, a mass compressing the spinal cord was identified, accompanied by yellowish fluid and moderate to severe spinal cord adhesions (**D**). However, culture studies of the yellowish pus in the postoperative state did not detect any specific bacteria or signs of infection (**E**), discontinuing the empirical antibiotics used initially.

3.4. Analysis of Revision Cases

In the seven revision cases, five were confirmed mass formations invading the spinal canal at least one month after surgery, with hematoma ruled out. These were categorized as the symptomatic spinal canal invasion group. They were further divided into BioGlue® and non-BioGlue® groups and underwent a simple t-test, which showed a statistically significant difference ($p = 0.001$) between the two groups. However, no statistically notable difference was found ($p = 0.080$) when the CSF leakage case was compared between the two groups (Table 2). Importantly, all seven revision surgeries occurred exclusively in the BioGlue® group. While only five of these were directly attributable to BioGlue®-associated mass formation, and the hematoma case was likely unrelated to BioGlue® use, the exclusive occurrence of all revision cases within the BioGlue® cohort may still warrant caution and further investigation regarding its clinical safety profile in intradural tumor surgery.

3.5. Logistic Regression Analysis for Risk Factors of ESCC Grades 2 and 3

We divided the 153 enrolled patients into ESCC grade 1, 2, and 3 groups to analyze the relationship between BioGlue® and ESCC grades from a different perspective. The univariate logistic analysis for ESCC grades 2 and 3 revealed that the use of BioGlue® had an OR of 3.931 with a p-value of 0.005, while Tachocomb® was not statistically significant with a p-value of 0.685. Furthermore, the cervical location was associated with an OR of 3.524 and a p-value of 0.047. A multivariate analysis was conducted on the categories with significant p-values and ORs in the univariate analysis, demonstrating an OR of 3.812 with a p-value = 0.003 for BioGlue®. On the other hand, cervical and thoracic locations had ORs less than 1, which was contrary to that observed in the univariate analysis: cervical location showed an OR of 0.196 with a p-value of 0.005, and thoracic location had an OR of 0.394 with a p-value of 0.107 (Table 4).

Table 4. Logistic regression analysis for ESCC Grades 2 and 3.

Variables	Univariable Analysis			Multivariable Analysis		
	OR	95% CI	p-Value	OR	95% CI	p-Value
Age (Ref.: below 70)						
≥70	2.571	0.907-7.290	0.076			
Sex (Ref.: Female)						
Male	2.060	0.815–5.209	0.127			
Location (Ref.: Lumbosacral)						
Cervical	3.524	1.018–12.197	0.047 *	0.196	0.063–0.610	0.005 *
Thoracic	1.764	0.505–6.164	0.374	0.394	0.127–1.224	0.107
Levels (Ref.: 1 level)						
2 levels	1.225	0.341–4.395	0.756			
≥3 levels	3.176	0.791–12.745	0.103			
Use of BioGlue®	3.931	1.514–10.212	0.005 **	3.812	1.570–9.258	0.003 **
Use of TachoComb®	1.340	0.327–5.499	0.685			

ESCC grade: epidural spinal cord compression scale; OR: odds ratio; CI: confidence intervals; Ref: reference; * $p < 0.05$; ** $p < 0.005$.

4. Discussion

This study identified a significant association between the use of BioGlue® and increased rates of postoperative mass formation, spinal canal invasion, and higher ESCC grades. Among 153 patients, most ESCC grade 2 or 3 cases were found in the BioGlue® group (Table 2). Notably, all five patients who underwent revision surgery for symptomatic spinal canal invasion belonged to the BioGlue® group (Table 3), and logistic regression analysis further confirmed BioGlue® as an independent predictor of higher ESCC grade (Table 4). These findings suggest that BioGlue® may contribute to a clinically significant mass effect following intradural tumor surgery.

Figure 2 presents a representative case in which a mass lesion persisted up to 9 months postoperatively and required surgical re-exploration. The lesion was clearly distinct from hematoma or tumor recurrence, and its MRI signal characteristics were consistent with previously reported BioGlue®-associated granulomas, or "Gluomas" [12]. Although causality cannot be definitively established, the consistency of imaging features, surgical findings, and their concordance with prior literature provides strong circumstantial evidence supporting this association.

Although all surgeries were performed by a single surgeon using a standardized thin layer application technique in accordance with published guidelines [14], mass formation still occurred in some patients. Intraoperative findings and negative culture results ruled out infectious etiologies in these compressive lesions, suggesting an alternative mechanism. This discrepancy between intended technique and adverse outcomes implies that factors beyond surgical application—such as localized anatomical constraints, pooling of adhesive, or individual tissue responses—may contribute to delayed BioGlue®-associated spinal canal invasion.

Widely used in cardiac surgery [1,2], BioGlue® has been extensively adopted in neurosurgery, including both cranial and spinal procedures, despite the manufacturer not providing assurances for its safety in spine surgery [4,6]. Various studies, including those by Miscusi et al., have concluded that BioGlue® in spine surgery is an effective adjunct to immediate dural repair in non-instrumented spinal surgery [3]. Its efficacy and safety were comparable to those of other sealants, potentially decreasing the incidence of associated short- and long-term complications. Yuen et al. reported a case demonstrating the persistence of BioGlue® at the repair site two years after its successful use in aiding dural closure during a lumbar decompressive procedure [5]. However, postoperative cases of gluoma formation causing a mass effect have also been reported. Rasul et al. described two cases where the use of BioGlue® caused a local reaction, forming a granuloma that led to cord compression several years after surgery [12]. Nonetheless, aside from such individual case reports, no case series or systematic research on this topic is available. Considering the factors mentioned above, our study is valuable in that it examines the long-term impacts of using BioGlue® and determines whether its application post-dural closure may cause spinal cord compression and neurological decline.

A previous study recognized BioGlue® as a low signal intensity on T2 MR images, thus differentiable from the CSF or other structures [17]; this aligned with our study findings that lesions caused a mass effect on the follow-up MRIs. However, the MRI findings for ESCC grade 2 or higher in the non-BioGlue® group were not clearly differentiated, posing difficulties in attributing the lesion to BioGlue®. While the epidural compressing lesions observed were likely to be hematomas in the non-BioGlue® group, they were not distinctive from BioGlue® in MRI.

Univariate logistic regression analysis also confirmed that surgery at a cervical location was associated with higher-grade ESCC. Such a relationship may be due to the smaller spinal canal in this region compared to the thoracic or lumbar levels, leading to more significant cord compression for the same mass effect [20–23]. Interestingly, this association was reversed in the multivariate analysis, where cervical location appeared to be a protective factor. While the application technique of BioGlue® was consistent across cases due to the use of a standardized thin-layer method by a single surgeon, we hypothesize that anatomical and procedural differences may account for this finding. Specifically, in cervical cases where laminoplasty was performed, the smaller size of cervical laminae and their reattachment with plates may have resulted in a relatively larger reconstructed spinal canal compared to thoracolumbar laminectomy. This increased canal dimension may have attenuated the mass effect of BioGlue®, resulting in a lower ESCC grade.

BioGlue® is known to cause toxic effects and wound infection as a side effect [9–11] in addition to the mass effect. The literature has anecdotally reported on the toxic effects of BioGlue®, associated with the possible development of aseptic meningitis due to the glutaraldehyde component. However, it is noteworthy that bovine serum albumin (45%) and glutaraldehyde (10%) are mixed in the applicator tip to form the glue, after which the glutaraldehyde no longer exists as a single component. While a prior study has demonstrated the biocompatibility of this sealant [24], it should be applied only extradurally with care. Furthermore, this study did not establish a clear connection between BioGlue® and wound infection but confirmed that all four patients with neurologic deterioration had lesions due to a mass effect, hence not identifying evidence to support the neurotoxicity or wound infection of BioGlue®.

This study had several limitations. First, its retrospective, non-randomized design introduces a risk of selection bias. Although all cases involved elective intradural tumor surgeries with intentional durotomies—reducing variability in the extent of dural defect—unmeasured confounding variables such as tumor morphology or dural fragility may have influenced the surgeon's decision to use BioGlue®. For example, dumbbell-shaped tumors requiring lateral dural incisions may have been more prone to CSF leakage and thus more likely to be treated with BioGlue®. Although all surgeries were performed by a single experienced surgeon using a standardized thin-layer application technique, the possibility of selection bias affecting outcomes cannot be completely excluded. Furthermore, while a prospective randomized controlled trial could better address these concerns, the potential risk of BioGlue®-associated mass effect observed in this study raises ethical concerns regarding the feasibility of such a design. Second, information was lacking on follow-up MRI for patients in the non-BioGlue® group with high-grade ESCC. Among the patients treated without BioGlue® and ESCC grades 2 and 3, only two showed resolutions of the lesion in follow-up MRI, limiting the ability to prove that the immediate post-surgical mass effects in patients not treated with BioGlue® are temporary and resolvable. Third, data on clinical symptoms such as pain or neurological deterioration were missing for patients with high-grade ESCC. Further studies should include changes in patients' clinical symptoms.

5. Conclusions

Our findings indicate that BioGlue® is a significant risk factor for mass formation aggravating spinal canal invasion after intradural spinal cord tumor surgery. Therefore, the use of BioGlue® to address CSF leakage in spine surgery is risky and should be limited.

Author Contributions: Conceptualization, J.H.P.; formal analysis, S.W.J.; investigation, S.W.J.; methodology, S.W.J. and J.H.P.; validation, J.H.P.; writing—original draft, S.W.J.; writing—review and editing, S.W.J., S.H.L., H.K.S., S.R.J., D.P., C.K. and J.H.P. All authors have read and agreed to the published version of the manuscript.

Funding: This research was supported by the Ulsan University Industry–University Cooperation Foundation under the project titled 'Cerebrospinal fluid (CSF) leakage prevention materials through animal studies', supported by Dalim Biotechnology Company, Limited (Project No. 2024-0454).

Institutional Review Board Statement: This study was conducted in accordance with Declaration of Helsinki and approved by the Institutional Review Board (IRB, No. 2023-1613, dated 21 December 2023), ensuring compliance with ethical standards.

Informed Consent Statement: Given the retrospective nature of the study, the IRB waived the requirement for informed consent.

Data Availability Statement: The raw data supporting the conclusions of this article will be made available by the authors on request.

Conflicts of Interest: None of the authors has any potential conflict of interest. The materials used in this study are not associated with Dalim Biotechnology Company, which provided the funding.

References

1. Passage, J.; Jalali, H.; Tam, R.K.; Harrocks, S.; O'Brien, M.F. BioGlue Surgical Adhesive—An appraisal of its indications in cardiac surgery. *Ann. Thorac. Surg.* **2002**, *74*, 432–437. [CrossRef] [PubMed]
2. Coselli, J.S.; Bavaria, J.E.; Fehrenbacher, J.; Stowe, C.L.; Macheers, S.K.; Gundry, S.R. Prospective randomized study of a protein-based tissue adhesive used as a hemostatic and structural adjunct in cardiac and vascular anastomotic repair procedures. *J. Am. Coll. Surg.* **2003**, *197*, 243–252. [CrossRef]
3. Miscusi, M.; Polli, F.M.; Forcato, S.; Coman, M.A.; Ricciardi, L.; Ramieri, A.; Raco, A. The use of surgical sealants in the repair of dural tears during non-instrumented spinal surgery. *Eur. Spine J.* **2014**, *23*, 1761–1766. [CrossRef] [PubMed]
4. Kumar, A.; Maartens, N.F.; Kaye, A.H. Reconstruction of the sellar floor using Bioglue following transsphenoidal procedures. *J. Clin. Neurosci.* **2003**, *10*, 92–95. [CrossRef]
5. Yuen, T.; Kaye, A.H. Persistence of Bioglue in spinal dural repair. *J. Clin. Neurosci.* **2005**, *12*, 100–101. [CrossRef] [PubMed]
6. Kumar, A.; Maartens, N.F.; Kaye, A.H. Evaluation of the use of BioGlue in neurosurgical procedures. *J. Clin. Neurosci.* **2003**, *10*, 661–664. [CrossRef]
7. Qiu, L.; Qi See, A.A.; Steele, T.W.J.; Kam King, N.K. Bioadhesives in neurosurgery: A review. *J. Neurosurg.* **2019**, *133*, 1928–1938. [CrossRef]
8. Epstein, N.E. Dural repair with four spinal sealants: Focused review of the manufacturers' inserts and the current literature. *Spine J.* **2010**, *10*, 1065–1068. [CrossRef]
9. Furst, W.; Banerjee, A. Release of glutaraldehyde from an albumin-glutaraldehyde tissue adhesive causes significant in vitro and in vivo toxicity. *Ann. Thorac. Surg.* **2005**, *79*, 1522–1528. [CrossRef]
10. Luthra, S.; Theodore, S.; Tatoulis, J. Bioglue: A word of caution. *Ann. Thorac. Surg.* **2008**, *86*, 1055–1056. [CrossRef]
11. Klimo, P., Jr.; Khalil, A.; Slotkin, J.R.; Smith, E.R.; Scott, R.M.; Goumnerova, L.C. Wound complications associated with the use of bovine serum albumin-glutaraldehyde surgical adhesive in pediatric patients. *Neurosurgery* **2007**, *60*, 305–309. [CrossRef] [PubMed]
12. Rasul, F.T.; Tusnea, D.; David, K.M. BioGlue(R) induced granuloma causing symptomatic spinal cord compression: A late complication. *Acta Neurochir.* **2018**, *160*, 195–198. [CrossRef] [PubMed]
13. Lauvin, M.A.; Zemmoura, I.; Cazals, X.; Cottier, J.P. Delayed cauda equina compression after spinal dura repair with BioGlue: Magnetic resonance imaging and computed tomography aspects of two cases of "glue-oma". *Spine J.* **2015**, *15*, e5–e8. [CrossRef] [PubMed]
14. Miscusi, M. BioGlue and spine surgery. *Spine J.* **2011**, *11*, 983. [CrossRef]
15. Braun, P.; Kazmi, K.; Nogues-Melendez, P.; Mas-Estelles, F.; Aparici-Robles, F. MRI findings in spinal subdural and epidural hematomas. *Eur. J. Radiol.* **2007**, *64*, 119–125. [CrossRef] [PubMed]
16. Holtas, S.; Heiling, M.; Lonntoft, M. Spontaneous spinal epidural hematoma: Findings at MR imaging and clinical correlation. *Radiology* **1996**, *199*, 409–413. [CrossRef]
17. Tarapore, P.E.; Mukherjee, P.; Mummaneni, P.V.; Ames, C.P. The appearance of dural sealants under MR imaging. *AJNR Am. J. Neuroradiol.* **2012**, *33*, 1530–1533. [CrossRef]
18. Altorfer, F.C.S.; Sutter, R.; Farshad, M.; Spirig, J.M.; Farshad-Amacker, N.A. MRI appearance of adjunct surgical material used in spine surgery. *Spine J.* **2022**, *22*, 75–83. [CrossRef]
19. Bilsky, M.H.; Laufer, I.; Fourney, D.R.; Groff, M.; Schmidt, M.H.; Varga, P.P.; Vrionis, F.D.; Yamada, Y.; Gerszten, P.C.; Kuklo, T.R. Reliability analysis of the epidural spinal cord compression scale. *J. Neurosurg. Spine* **2010**, *13*, 324–328. [CrossRef]
20. Morishita, Y.; Naito, M.; Hymanson, H.; Miyazaki, M.; Wu, G.; Wang, J.C. The relationship between the cervical spinal canal diameter and the pathological changes in the cervical spine. *Eur. Spine J.* **2009**, *18*, 877–883. [CrossRef]
21. Edwards, W.C.; LaRocca, S.H. The developmental segmental sagittal diameter in combined cervical and lumbar spondylosis. *Spine* **1985**, *10*, 42–49. [CrossRef] [PubMed]
22. Hayashi, H.; Okada, K.; Hamada, M.; Tada, K.; Ueno, R. Etiologic factors of myelopathy. A radiographic evaluation of the aging changes in the cervical spine. *Clin. Orthop. Relat. Res.* **1987**, *214*, 200–209. [CrossRef]
23. Torg, J.S.; Naranja, R.J., Jr.; Pavlov, H.; Galinat, B.J.; Warren, R.; Stine, R.A. The relationship of developmental narrowing of the cervical spinal canal to reversible and irreversible injury of the cervical spinal cord in football players. *J. Bone Jt. Surg. Am.* **1996**, *78*, 1308–1314. [CrossRef]
24. Stylli, S.S.; Kumar, A.; Gonzales, M.; Kaye, A.H. The biocompatibility of BioGlue with the cerebral cortex: A pilot study. *J. Clin. Neurosci.* **2004**, *11*, 631–635. [CrossRef] [PubMed]

Journal of
Clinical Medicine

MDPI

Article

Clinical Significance of Prognostic Nutritional Index in Patients Who Underwent Palliative Surgery for Spine Metastasis

Young-Hoon Kim [1], Kee-Yong Ha [1], Hyung-Youl Park [2], Kihyun Kwon [1], Yunseong Kim [1], Hyun W. Bae [3] and Sang-Il Kim [1,*]

1 Department of Orthopedic Surgery, Seoul St. Mary's Hospital, College of Medicine, The Catholic University of Korea, Seoul 06591, Republic of Korea; boscoa@catholic.ac.kr (Y.-H.K.); kyh@catholic.ac.kr (K.-Y.H.); 899835@naver.com (K.K.); cinar@naver.com (Y.K.)
2 Department of Orthopedic Surgery, Eunpyeong St. Mary's Hospital, College of Medicine, The Catholic University of Korea, Seoul 03312, Republic of Korea; matrixbest@naver.com
3 Department of Orthopedic Surgery, Cedars-Sinai Medical Center, Los Angeles, CA 90048, USA; baemd@me.com
* Correspondence: sang1kim81@gmail.com

Abstract: Background/Objectives: Malnutrition is common in patients with metastatic spine tumors (MSTs) and may adversely affect surgical outcomes. The Prognostic Nutritional Index (PNI) reflects both nutritional and immune status, but its role in palliative MST surgery is not well defined. The aim of this study was to investigate the association between preoperative the PNI and postoperative outcomes, including functional recovery and survival, in patients undergoing palliative surgery for MSTs. **Methods**: A brief description of the main methods or treatments applied. This can include any relevant preregistration or specimen information. **Results**: Patients with a higher PNI ($\geq$42.8) demonstrated significantly better postoperative ambulation and longer overall survival compared to those with a lower PNI (<42.8). The higher PNI group showed earlier ambulation ($p = 0.017$) and longer median survival (30.7 vs. 7.0 months; $p = 0.002$). Multivariate analysis confirmed that a PNI $\geq$ 42.8 was an independent predictor of early ambulation (HR = 1.516; 95% CI: 1.010–2.277; $p = 0.045$) and prolonged survival (HR = 0.955; 95% CI: 0.927–0.985; $p = 0.003$). No significant association was found between the PNI and postoperative infections. **Conclusions**: The PNI is a simple and effective predictor of postoperative functional recovery and survival in patients undergoing palliative surgery for MSTs. Its routine preoperative assessment may help stratify surgical risk, guide nutritional interventions, and optimize clinical outcomes in this vulnerable population.

Keywords: spine metastasis; palliative surgery; nutrition; prognostic nutritional index; ambulatory function; survival

1. Introduction

A recent epidemiological study reported that approximately 23 million people had cancer in 2019, which was 2.3 times than in 1990 [1]. Bone is the most common site for the metastases of many cancers. Most cancers often metastasize to the axial skeleton, with the spine being the most frequent site of bone metastasis, accounting for 87% [2,3]. Although not all spine metastases will have clinical manifestations, symptomatic spine metastasis can cause pain, neurological deficits, and even the loss of ambulatory function, leading to increased mortality and decreased quality of life [4,5]. The treatment goal for metastatic spine tumors (MSTs) is predominantly palliative to reduce pain and to preserve or improve neurologic status [4,5]. It has been reported that the surgical treatment for

MSTs has increased over the past few decades [6,7]. Surgical treatment can influence subsequent additional cancer treatment and even overall survival [8,9]. Although surgical techniques have improved, postoperative complications are quite common after surgical treatment for MSTs because cancer patients are usually frail and malnourished with medical comorbidities and poor functional status [10].

Malnutrition is a common disorder in cancer patients, accounting for 40%, especially in those with advanced stages [11,12]. Although the pathophysiology of malnutrition is complex, it is mainly a consequence of inadequate food intake caused by cancer itself or side effects during anticancer treatment in cancer patients [13]. Besides starvation-type malnutrition, there is another type of malnutrition called inflammation-type malnutrition, in which systemic inflammation increases due to metabolic derangement. Both types of malnutrition can put patients at greater risk of poorer adverse events, such as increased morbidity, complications, length of stay, and even mortality [14,15].

Various scoring tools are available to assess nutritional status such as the Mini Nutritional Assessment, Prognostic Nutritional Index (PNI), and Nutritional Risk Index (NRI). The PNI is calculated using serum albumin and lymphocyte count, which make it easier to use than other metrics [16]. The serum albumin level is a widely used indicator for nutritional status and disease status of cancer patients [17]. Lymphocyte count is reflective of inflammatory status. Elevated systemic inflammation in cancer patients is associated with poor prognosis and the development of inflammation-type malnutrition [18]. Recent studies have found that the PNI has significant prognostic value in cancer treatment [19–22].

Despite growing evidence supporting the utility of the PNI in oncology, its role in the specific context of palliative surgery for MSTs remains underexplored. Given that functional recovery and quality of life are primary goals in this population, identifying reliable preoperative prognostic markers is essential. Moreover, considering the high prevalence of malnutrition in patients with MSTs, preoperative nutritional assessment using the PNI could help stratify surgical risk and guide perioperative management. Therefore, this study aimed to investigate the association between the preoperative PNI and postoperative outcomes, including functional recovery and overall survival, in patients undergoing palliative surgery for MSTs. By elucidating this relationship, we hope to provide evidence that supports the integration of nutritional assessment into preoperative risk stratification and clinical decision making in this vulnerable patient population.

2. Materials and Methods

2.1. Patient Selection

This study was approved by the Institutional Review Board of our institute (approval No. KC24RISI0293, approval date 7 May 2024). This retrospective study used prospectively collected data for all patients who underwent spine surgery for MSTs in a tertiary single institute from January 2017 to June 2021. During the study period, 195 patients underwent spine surgery for MSTs in our institute. Inclusion criteria were as follows: age of more than 18 years, palliative debulking surgery, and preoperative preservation of independent ambulatory function. If the surgery was performed to relieve preoperative symptoms caused by a metastatic spine tumor but was not intended as a curative excision, the authors defined it as "palliative debulking surgery." We adapted the Nurick grading system to evaluate ambulatory function [23]. If the patient showed a Nurick grade 4 or higher (able to walk with an aid), we determined that the patient was ambulatory. Exclusion criteria were as follows: preoperative Nurick grade 5 (chair-bound or bedridden), curative surgery, any preoperative nutritional interventions, revision surgery at the index level, lack of data, or follow-up period of less than 30 days after surgery.

2.2. Data Collection

We recorded clinical and surgical data. Patient data included age, sex, and body mass index (BMI). Clinical data included American Society of Anesthesiologists (ASA) classification, Eastern Cooperative Oncology Group (ECOG) performance status, primary cancer, history of oncological treatment (chemotherapy or radiotherapy), and modified Charlson Comorbidity Index (mCCI) [24]. Because all patients had cancer, the mCCI was calculated with the exclusion of 6 points for cancer. Surgery-related data included the length of operated segments, estimated blood loss (EBL), use of instrumentation, and need for intensive care unit (ICU). PNI was calculated with the following formula: 10 $\times$ serum albumin (g/dL) + 0.005 $\times$ total lymphocyte count (/mm^3) [16]. Currently, there is no consensus on the normal range of PNI. Thus, we divided patients into two groups and compared them based on the mean PNI value of our cohort. Perioperative complications including surgical site infection and other infectious conditions (e.g., pneumonia, cellulitis) were investigated. Surgical site infection (SSI) (either superficial or deep) was diagnosed based on the definition of the Centers for Disease Control and Prevention [25]. Postoperative times to start ambulation and postoperative survival were reviewed.

2.3. Statistical Analysis

All statistical analyses were performed using SPSS software (IBM SPSS Statistics for Windows, v24; IBM Corp., Sydney NSW, Australia). Continuous variables are expressed as mean and standard deviation, and they were analyzed with unpaired *t*-test. Categorical variables are expressed as absolute numbers and percentages, and they were analyzed with chi-square test or Fisher's exact test as appropriate. Survivorship was subjected to Kaplan–Meier analysis. Log-rank test was used to compare outcomes between groups. Cox proportional hazard models were used to analyze the correlation between PNI and postoperative ambulatory function or survival. Receiver operating characteristic (ROC) analysis was performed for postoperative ambulatory function and overall survival. For all analyses, p values of less than 0.05 were considered significant.

3. Results

3.1. Preoperative and Operative Details

Among 195 patients who underwent surgery during the study period, a total of 133 patients met the criteria and were included in this study (Figure 1). Baseline demographic and oncological details of these 133 patients are shown in Table 1. Of these patients, 78 (58.6%) were male. The mean age was 61.1 years for the 133 patients included in this study. The preoperative mean BMI was 23.0 $\pm$ 3.3 kg/m^2, the mean mCCI was 7.1 $\pm$ 1.3, and the mean PNI was 42.8 $\pm$ 7.5. The mean postoperative follow-up period was 15.8 $\pm$ 14.1 months. Multiple myeloma (n = 35) and lung cancer (n = 34) were the most common primary cancers, followed by breast cancer (n = 13). Perioperative data are summarized in Table 2. A total of 119 patients underwent instrumented surgery, and the remaining 14 patients underwent decompression surgery without instrumentation. The mean number of operated levels was 3.8 $\pm$ 1.7 for instrumented surgery and 1.9 $\pm$ 1.0 for decompression only. Mean perioperative blood loss was 906.6 $\pm$ 815.9 mL, and postoperative ICU care was needed for 44 patients (33.1%). Mean values of serum albumin level and lymphocyte count were 3.7 $\pm$ 0.6 g/dL and 1215 $\pm$ 590/mm^3, respectively. The mean PNI was 42.8 $\pm$ 7.5.

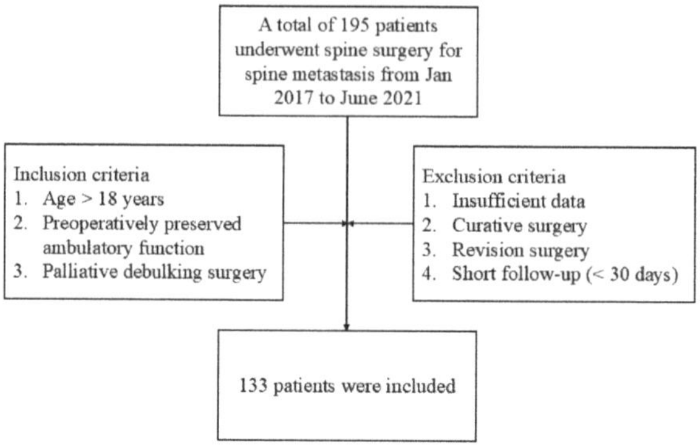

Figure 1. Flow chart for inclusion and exclusion.

Table 1. Baseline demographic and oncological data (divided into two groups according to mean PNI [42.8]).

	Total (n = 133)	**102 Patients Who Could Walk Independently After Surgery**		
		PNI ≥ 42.8 (n = 59)	**PNI < 42.8 (n = 43)**	p
Age (years)	61.1 ± 12.2	57.7 ± 11.9	62.8 ± 12.0	0.037 #
Male	58.6% (n = 78)	61.0% (n = 36)	53.5% (n = 23)	0.543 *
Body mass index (kg/m^2)	23.0 ± 3.3	22.8 ± 3.0	22.8 ± 3.9	0.927 #
Primary cancer				0.147 ***
Multiple myeloma	35	13	15	
Lung cancer	34	15	9	
Breast cancer	13	9	2	
Prostate cancer	10	3	3	
Others	39	19	14	
Prior chemotherapy	54.1% (n = 72)	54.2% (n = 32)	44.2% (n = 19)	0.423 *
Prior radiotherapy at index level	12.8% (n = 17)	11.9% (n = 7)	9.3% (n = 4)	0.757 **
Modified Charlson comorbidity index	7.1 ±1.3	6.7 ± 1.0	7.5 ± 1.4	0.001 #
ASA classification				0.002 ***
II	47	28	9	
III	71	29	28	
IV	15	2	6	
ECOG				0.140 ***
0	17	10	5	
1	59	29	19	
2	46	18	14	
3	11	2	5	
Serum albumin level (g/dL)	3.7 ± 0.6	4.1 ± 0.4	3.3 ± 0.4	<0.001 #
Lymphocyte count (/mL)	1215 ± 590	1404 ± 479	1002 ± 435	<0.001 #
Prognostic nutritional index	42.8 ± 7.5	48.4 ± 4.0	37.3 ± 4.1	<0.001 #

Independent *t*-test for #, chi-square test for *, Fisher's exact test for **, and linear-by-linear test for *** were used.

Table 2. Perioperative data (divided into two groups according to mean PNI [42.8]).

	Total (n = 133)	102 Patients Who Could Walk Independently After Surgery		
		PNI ≥ 42.8 (n = 59)	PNI < 42.8 (n = 43)	p
Surgery type With instrumentation Without instrumentation	 89.5% (n = 119) 10.5% (n = 14)	 84.7% (n = 50) 15.3% (n = 9)	 97.7% (n = 42) 2.3% (n = 1)	0.042 *
Number of instrumented levels	3.8 ± 1.7	3.6 ± 1.7	3.5 ± 1.5	0.665 #
Blood loss (mL)	906.6 ± 815.9	773.3 ± 809.2	1046.8 ± 901.4	0.118 #
ICU care	33.1% (n = 44)	32.2% (n = 19)	23.3% (n = 10)	0.323 *

Independent t-test for # and chi-square test for * were used.

3.2. Relationship Between PNI and Infection

SSI was identified in 10 patients (7.5%). Comparing patients with and without SSI, there was no significant difference in the PNI between the two groups (39.5 ± 6.2 vs. 43.1 ± 7.6, p = 0.148). Infectious conditions other than SSI occurred in 13 patients (9.8%). Comparing patients with and without infectious conditions, there was no significant difference in the PNI between the two groups either (41.1 ± 11.5 vs. 43.0 ± 7.0, p = 0.568) (Table 3).

Table 3. Relationship between the Prognostic Nutritional Index (PNI) and the occurrence of infectious conditions.

	Surgical Site Infections		Other Infections	
	Yes (n = 10)	No (n = 123)	Yes (n = 13)	No (n = 120)
PNI value	39.5 ± 6.2	43.1 ± 7.6	41.1 ± 11.5	43.0 ± 7.0
p	0.148		0.568	

Independent t-test was used.

3.3. Relationship Between PNI and Ambulatory Function

At postoperative 1 month, 102 patients (77.3%) showed ambulatory function. They had a higher preoperative PNI than 30 patients with the loss of ambulatory function (43.7 ± 6.8 vs. 39.6 ± 9.1, p = 0.008). We performed a sub-analysis for 102 patients with postoperative ambulatory function. When analyzing two groups divided based on the mean value of the PNI (42.8), patients with a higher PNI (≥42.8) showed earlier ambulatory function after surgery than those with a lower PNI on the log-rank test (p = 0.017) (Figure 2). In the multivariate Cox biohazard model, a PNI greater than 42.8 was a significantly positive factor for earlier postoperative ambulation (HR = 1.516; 95% CI = 1.010–2.277; p = 0.045). The ROC curve for ambulatory function at postoperative 1 month is shown in Figure 3. Area under the curve (AUC) was 0.642, and the optimal cut-off value of the PNI was 36.1 (sensitivity = 0.863, specificity = 0.419).

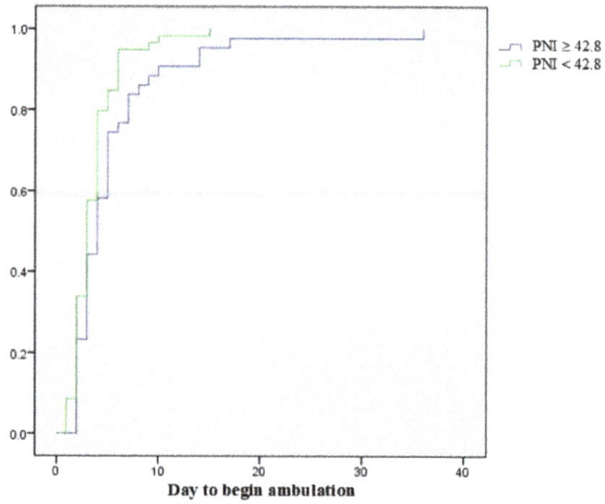

Figure 2. Log-rank test shows that patients with a PNI higher than 42.8 show earlier ambulatory function after surgery than those with a PNI less than 42.8 ($p = 0.017$).

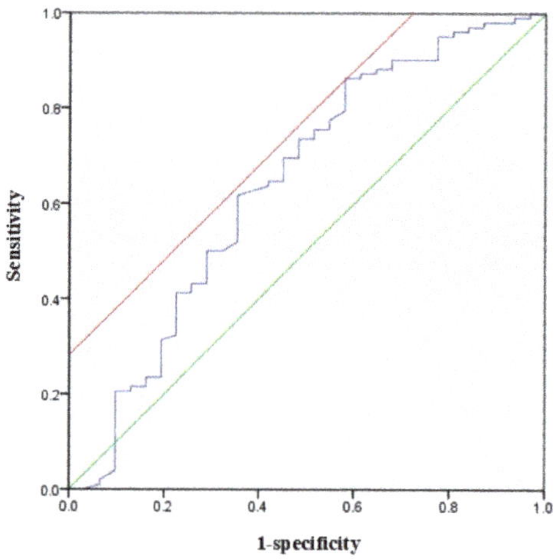

Figure 3. ROC curve for ambulatory function at postoperative 1 month. A green line indicates the diagonal reference line and a red line indicates the a tangent representing the Youden index for the optimal cutoff point.

3.4. PNI and Postoperative Survival

Median overall survival of all patients was 540 days. Mortality rates at 3 months and 12 months were 81.6% and 57.1%, respectively. A log-rank test demonstrated that patients with a PNI higher than 42.8 had longer median overall survival (30.7 months; 95% CI 15.9–45.5 months) than those with a PNI lower than 42.8 (7 months; 95% CI 1.1–13.2 months, $p = 0.002$) (Figure 4). A lower PNI (< 42.8) was associated with a significantly lower median overall survival (HR = 0.955; 95% CI = 0.927–0.985; $p = 0.003$). The ROC curve for overall survival at postoperative 3 months is shown in Figure 5. The area under the curve (AUC) was 0.688, and the optimal cut-off value of the PNI was 42.0 (sensitivity = 0.648, specificity = 0.714).

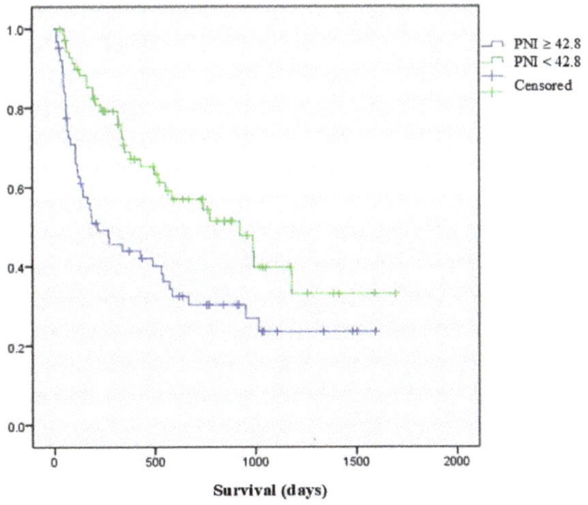

Figure 4. Log-rank test shows that patients with a PNI higher than 42.8 have longer overall survival (median of 30.7 months; 95% CI for 15.9–45.5 months) than those with a PNI lower than 42.8 (median of 7 months; 95% CI for 1.1–13.2 months; $p = 0.002$).

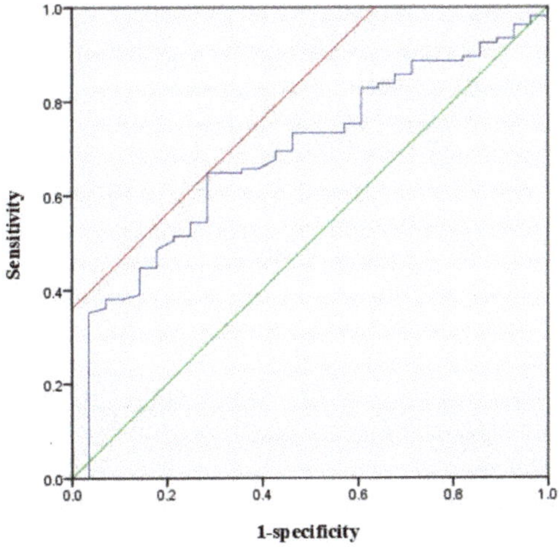

Figure 5. ROC curve for overall survival at postoperative 1 month. A green line indicates the diagonal reference line and a red line indicates the a tangent representing the Youden index for the optimal cutoff point.

4. Discussion

The PNI, which consists of nutritional (serum albumin level) and immunological (lymphocyte count) indices, is widely used as a predictive indicator of postoperative morbidities and mortality in cancer patients [19–22]. This study investigated the prognostic significance of the preoperative PNI in patients undergoing palliative surgery for MSTs. Our findings demonstrate that a lower PNI is significantly associated with delayed postoperative ambulation and decreased overall survival. Although the PNI was not significantly associated with postoperative infections, its correlations with functional and survival outcomes underscore its clinical value. The PNI, derived from serum albumin and lymphocyte count, reflects both nutritional status and systemic immune function. Patients with a PNI $\geq$ 42.8 were more likely to achieve early ambulation. They had a median overall survival of

30.7 months, higher than a median overall survival of 7.0 months for patients with a lower PNI. These results are clinically meaningful, particularly in the context of palliative surgery, where functional recovery and quality of life are primary goals.

The possible relationship between a low PNI and impaired ambulatory recovery likely reflects underlying sarcopenia. Although we did not directly measure skeletal muscle mass, sarcopenia and malnutrition often coexist in advanced cancer, particularly under chronic systemic inflammation [26,27]. Our recent study has found that both the PNI and the psoas muscle index are independent predictors of postoperative recovery and complication risk in MST surgery [28]. Similarly, Ushiku et al. have demonstrated that skeletal muscle mass assessed by total psoas area (TPA)/vertebral body area can predict short-term postoperative function [29]. These studies highlighted the synergistic impact of nutrition and muscle mass on surgical outcomes. However, given the absence of direct sarcopenia assessment in our cohort, these interpretations should be considered exploratory and serve as a basis for future prospective research.

In recent decades, there has been important progress in radiotherapy (RT) for cancer treatment [30]. RT is effective for pain reduction and local tumor control. Recent studies showed that sarcopenia or malnutrition did not seem to affect treatment outcomes and complications after radiotherapy in bladder cancer patients [31,32]. Therefore, RT may be a more appropriate option, especially in patients with poor prognostic predictors, such as a low PNI.

Our findings on survival were also consistent with previous studies. Iinuma et al. have proposed a PNI cutoff of $\geq$42.5 as a significant predictor of 6-month survival, closely matching the mean value in our cohort [33]. This reinforces the use of the PNI as an objective, prognostically relevant preoperative marker. Ramos et al. have compared six nutritional biomarkers—the PNI, NRI, Controlling Nutritional Status Score (CONUT), TPA, BMI, and body weight—for predicting mortality and wound complications after MST surgery [34]. They found that the PNI, NRI, and CONUT had the highest discriminatory power for 90-day and 12-month mortality (c-statistics: 0.74–0.75) and that each biomarker predicted survival independently of performance status and tumor type. Interestingly, commonly used biomarkers BMI and TPA showed lower predictive accuracies, emphasizing the superior prognostic value of composite indices such as the PNI.

Although we did not find a significant association between the PNI and postoperative infections in our cohort, it is important to interpret this in the context of broader evidence. A possible explanation might be the relatively low overall incidence of SSI in our study population or the presence of multiple contributing surgical and patient-level risk factors beyond nutrition. However, extensive evidence supports a strong link between malnutrition and postoperative infection. For instance, Tsantes et al. have conducted a meta-analysis of 22 studies including over 175,000 patients and found that malnourished patients are more than twice as likely to develop SSI following a spinal surgery (OR 2.31; 95% CI 1.75–3.05) [35]. This study underscores the clinical importance of identifying and addressing malnutrition preoperatively to reduce preventable complications. While the PNI did not correlate with infection in our analysis, its roles in inflammatory and immune responses highlight its potential as part of a broader perioperative infection risk stratification.

Beyond statistical performance, Ramos et al. have advocated for the routine incorporation of the PNI and related markers into surgical decision making, particularly because their predictive value is comparable to, or even better than, some traditional prognostic scoring systems (e.g., Tokuhashi, Tomita, Bauer) [34]. This supports our position that preoperative nutritional status should be used not only to stratify risk but also to guide preoperative optimization. Additionally, Rigney et al. have emphasized that formal preoperative nutrition consultation can reduce wound-related complications and overall morbidity after MST surgery [36]. These findings highlight the modifiable nature of malnutrition and suggest that early nutritional interventions might yield measurable improvements in surgical outcomes.

This study has several limitations. First, the retrospective design introduced potential selection bias and limited causal interpretation. Although this study was based on prospectively collected data, unmeasured confounders such as comorbidities, psychosocial factors, and/or variations in nutrition and activity might have affected outcomes. Second, the single-center setting at a tertiary hospital might reduce generalizability to other institutions with different patient demographics or perioperative protocols. We used the mean PNI value from our cohort for analysis, which may limit the generalizability of our findings. In a previous report, a PNI cutoff of ≥42.9 was suggested as a predictor of better performance status. However, multi-institutional studies are needed to establish a standardized cutoff for the PNI in the future. Third, we used the PNI as a sole nutritional marker. While convenient and validated, it does not account for muscle mass or strength, although both muscle mass and strength are core elements of sarcopenia. We could not directly assess sarcopenia in this study, although it is likely to affect ambulatory function. Also, the reliability of the PNI could be compromised in patients with certain tumor types, such as hepatocellular carcinoma, typically associated with hypoalbuminemia [37]. Fourth, although the PNI is potentially modifiable, we did not evaluate whether nutritional interventions before surgery improved functional or survival outcomes. Fifth, our results about postoperative infection could be a type II error due to its low incidence. Previous reports showed that malnourished patients are more than twice as likely to develop SSI following spine surgery. Finally, because our cohort excluded non-ambulatory patients preoperatively, our findings might not be applicable to those with severe neurological deficits or poor performance status, nor to patients undergoing nonoperative or minimally invasive treatments.

While our study demonstrated the prognostic significance of the PNI in predicting postoperative ambulatory function and overall survival, we acknowledge that its application in routine clinical practice could be further enhanced through the development of a nomogram that integrates the PNI with other relevant clinical variables. Additionally, bioinformatic approaches could be employed to refine predictive models and identify novel biomarkers associated with outcomes in MST patients. Future studies should aim to establish such models prospectively to improve risk stratification and individualized patient counseling. Also, future research should focus on integrating nutritional and sarcopenic metrics into comprehensive prognostic models and testing whether nutritional or multimodal prehabilitation strategies can improve the outcomes of MST surgery. Given the growing body of literature, randomized trials evaluating perioperative nutritional supplementation, such as those described in recent lumbar surgery studies, might be warranted in the spine oncology population.

5. Conclusions

The PNI is a powerful, cost-effective biomarker that can independently predict functional recovery and the survival of patients undergoing palliative spine surgery. Its clinical utility is reinforced by growing evidence from recent studies comparing nutritional biomarkers in MST. Given its prognostic robustness and ease of use, the PNI should be integrated into standard preoperative evaluation to support risk stratification, patient counseling, and perioperative planning in this vulnerable patient population.

Author Contributions: Conceptualization, S.-I.K., H.W.B., and Y.-H.K.; methodology, Y.K.; formal analysis, K.-Y.H. and H.-Y.P.; investigation, S.-I.K. and H.-Y.P.; data curation, K.K.; writing—original draft preparation, S.-I.K.; writing—review and editing, S.-I.K. and K.-Y.H.; supervision, Y.-H.K. All authors have read and agreed to the published version of the manuscript.

Funding: This research received no external funding.

Institutional Review Board Statement: This study was conducted in accordance with the Declaration of Helsinki and approved by the Institutional Review Board of Seoul St. Mary's Hospital (KC24RISI0293, approval date 7 May 2024).

Informed Consent Statement: Patient consent was waived due to retrospective study design.

Data Availability Statement: Original data will be made available upon reasonable request.

Conflicts of Interest: The authors declare no conflicts of interest.

Abbreviations

The following abbreviations are used in this manuscript:

MST	Metastatic spine tumor
NRI	Nutritional risk index
PNI	Prognostic nutritional index
SSI	Surgical site infection
BMI	Body mass index
ASA	American Society of Anesthesiologists
ECOG	Eastern Cooperative Oncology Group
mCCI	Modified Charlson Comorbidity Index
EBL	Estimated blood loss
ICU	Intensive care unit
TPA	Total psoas area

References

1. Lin, L.; Li, Z.; Yan, L.; Liu, Y.; Yang, H.; Li, H. Global, regional, and national cancer incidence and death for 29 cancer groups in 2019 and trends analysis of the global cancer burden, 1990–2019. *J. Hematol. Oncol.* **2021**, *14*, 1–24. [CrossRef] [PubMed]
2. Coleman, R.E.; Croucher, P.I.; Padhani, A.R.; Clézardin, P.; Chow, E.; Fallon, M.; Guise, T.; Colangeli, S.; Capanna, R.; Costa, L. Bone metastases. *Nat. Rev. Dis. Prim.* **2020**, *6*, 1–28. [CrossRef]
3. Boxer, D.I.; Todd, C.E.; Coleman, R.; Fogelman, I. Bone secondaries in breast cancer: The solitary metastasis. *J. Nucl. Medicine.* **1989**, *30*, 1318–1320.
4. Hong, S.H.; Chang, B.-S.; Kim, H.; Kang, D.-H.; Chang, S.Y. An Updated Review on the Treatment Strategy for Spinal Metastasis from the Spine Surgeon's Perspective. *Asian Spine J.* **2022**, *16*, 799–811. [CrossRef] [PubMed]
5. Chang, S.Y.; Mok, S.; Park, S.C.; Kim, H.; Chang, B.-S. Treatment Strategy for Metastatic Spinal Tumors: A Narrative Review. *Asian Spine J.* **2020**, *14*, 513–525. [CrossRef]
6. Yoshihara, H.; Yoneoka, D. Trends in the surgical treatment for spinal metastasis and the in-hospital patient outcomes in the United States from 2000 to 2009. *Spine J.* **2014**, *14*, 1844–1849. [CrossRef]
7. Luksanapruksa, P.; Santipas, B.; Ruangchainikom, M.; Korwutthikulrangsri, E.; Pichaisak, W.; Wilartratsami, S. Epidemiologic Study of Operative Treatment for Spinal Metastasis in Thailand: A Review of National Healthcare Data from 2005 to 2014. *J. Korean Neurosurg. Soc.* **2022**, *65*, 57–63. [CrossRef]
8. Leitner, L.; Bratschitsch, G.; Kostwein, A.; Sadoghi, P.; Smolle, M.; Leithner, A.; Posch, F. More help than harm: Surgery for metastatic spinal cord compression is associated with more favorable overall survival within a propensity score analysis. *Eur. Spine J.* **2023**, *32*, 2468–2478. [CrossRef]
9. Zaborovskii, N.; Schlauch, A.; Shapton, J.; Denisov, A.; Ptashnikov, D.; Mikaylov, D.; Masevnin, S.; Smekalenkov, O.; Murakhovsky, V.; Kondrashov, D. Conditional survival after surgery for metastatic tumors of the spine: Does prognosis change over time? *Eur. Spine J.* **2023**, *32*, 1010–1020. [CrossRef]
10. Tarawneh, A.M.; Pasku, D.; Quraishi, N.A. Surgical complications and re-operation rates in spinal metastases surgery: A systematic review. *Eur. Spine J.* **2020**, *30*, 2791–2799. [CrossRef]
11. Marshall, K.M.; Loeliger, J.; Nolte, L.; Kelaart, A.; Kiss, N.K. Prevalence of malnutrition and impact on clinical outcomes in cancer services: A comparison of two time points. *Clin. Nutr.* **2019**, *38*, 644–651. [CrossRef] [PubMed]
12. Riad, A.; Knight, S.R.; Ghosh, D.; Kingsley, P.A.; Lapitan, M.C.; Parreno-Sacdalan, M.D.; Sundar, S.; Qureshi, A.U.; Valparaiso, A.P.; Pius, R.; et al. Impact of malnutrition on early outcomes after cancer surgery: An international, multicentre, prospective cohort study. *Lancet Glob. Health* **2023**, *11*, e341–e349. [CrossRef] [PubMed]

13. Arends, J. Malnutrition in cancer patients: Causes, consequences and treatment options. *Eur. J. Surg. Oncol. (EJSO)* **2023**, *50*, 107074. [CrossRef]
14. Tan, C.S.Y.; Read, J.A.; Phan, V.H.; Beale, P.J.; Peat, J.K.; Clarke, S.J. The relationship between nutritional status, inflammatory markers and survival in patients with advanced cancer: A prospective cohort study. *Support. Care Cancer* **2014**, *23*, 385–391. [CrossRef]
15. Mantzorou, M.; Koutelidakis, A.; Theocharis, S.; Giaginis, C. Clinical Value of Nutritional Status in Cancer: What is its Impact and how it Affects Disease Progression and Prognosis? *Nutr. Cancer* **2017**, *69*, 1151–1176. [CrossRef]
16. Buzby, G.P.; Mullen, J.L.; Matthews, D.C.; Hobbs, C.L.; Rosato, E.F. Prognostic nutritional index in gastrointestinal surgery. *Am. J. Surg.* **1980**, *139*, 160–167. [CrossRef]
17. Gupta, D.; Lis, C.G. Pretreatment serum albumin as a predictor of cancer survival: A systematic review of the epidemiological literature. *Nutr. J.* **2010**, *9*, 69. [CrossRef] [PubMed]
18. Mangano, G.D.; Fouani, M.; D'amico, D.; Di Felice, V.; Barone, R. Cancer-Related Cachexia: The Vicious Circle between Inflammatory Cytokines, Skeletal Muscle, Lipid Metabolism and the Possible Role of Physical Training. *Int. J. Mol. Sci.* **2022**, *23*, 3004. [CrossRef]
19. Li, J.; Zhu, N.; Wang, C.; You, L.; Guo, W.; Yuan, Z.; Qi, S.; Zhao, H.; Yu, J.; Huang, Y. Preoperative albumin-to-globulin ratio and prognostic nutritional index predict the prognosis of colorectal cancer: A retrospective study. *Sci. Rep.* **2023**, *13*, 1–15. [CrossRef]
20. Okadome, K.; Baba, Y.M.; Yagi, T.; Kiyozumi, Y.; Ishimoto, T.M.; Iwatsuki, M.M.; Miyamoto, Y.M.; Yoshida, N.M.; Watanabe, M.M.; Baba, H.M. Prognostic Nutritional Index, Tumor-infiltrating Lymphocytes, and Prognosis in Patients with Esophageal Cancer. *Ann. Surg.* **2020**, *271*, 693–700. [CrossRef]
21. Wang, B.; Zhang, J.; Shi, Y.; Wang, Y. Clinical significance of the combined systemic immune-inflammatory index and prognostic nutritional index in predicting the prognosis of patients with extensive-stage small-cell lung cancer receiving immune-combination chemotherapy. *BMC Cancer* **2024**, *24*, 1574. [CrossRef] [PubMed]
22. Yang, Y.; Gao, P.; Song, Y.; Sun, J.; Chen, X.; Zhao, J.; Ma, B.; Wang, Z. The prognostic nutritional index is a predictive indicator of prognosis and postoperative complications in gastric cancer: A meta-analysis. *Eur. J. Surg. Oncol. (EJSO)* **2016**, *42*, 1176–1182. [CrossRef] [PubMed]
23. Nurjck, S. The pathogenesis of the spinal cord disorder associated with cervical spondylosis. *Brain* **1972**, *95*, 87–100. [CrossRef] [PubMed]
24. Charlson, M.E.; Pompei, P.; Ales, K.L.; MacKenzie, C.R. A new method of classifying prognostic comorbidity in longitudinal studies: Development and validation. *J. Chronic Dis.* **1987**, *40*, 373–383. [CrossRef]
25. Borchardt, R.A.P.-C.; Tzizik, D.M. Update on surgical site infections: The new CDC guidelines. *J. Am. Acad. Physician Assist.* **2018**, *31*, 52–54. [CrossRef]
26. Jain, R.; Coss, C.; Whooley, P.; Phelps, M.; Owen, D.H. The Role of Malnutrition and Muscle Wasting in Advanced Lung Cancer. *Curr. Oncol. Rep.* **2020**, *22*, 1–10. [CrossRef]
27. Bossi, P.; Delrio, P.; Mascheroni, A.; Zanetti, M. The Spectrum of Malnutrition/Cachexia/Sarcopenia in Oncology According to Different Cancer Types and Settings: A Narrative Review. *Nutrients* **2021**, *13*, 1980. [CrossRef]
28. Bang, C.; Ko, M.-S.; Ko, Y.-I.; Kim, Y.-H. Effects of sarcopenia and nutritional status on surgical outcomes for metastatic spinal tumors: In the perspective of peri-operative complications and performance improvement. *Acta Neurochir.* **2024**, *166*, 423. [CrossRef]
29. Ushiku, C.; Akiyama, S.; Ikegami, T.; Inoue, T.; Shinohara, A.; Kobayashi, S.; Kajiwara, T.; Arimura, D.; Katsumi, S.; Obata, S.; et al. Clinical study of preoperative skeletal muscle mass as a predictor of physical performance recovery following palliative surgery for spinal metastases. *J. Orthop. Sci.* **2022**, *28*, 874–879. [CrossRef]
30. Giammalva, G.R.; Ferini, G.; Torregrossa, F.; Brunasso, L.; Musso, S.; Benigno, U.E.; Gerardi, R.M.; Bonosi, L.; Costanzo, R.; Paolini, F.; et al. The Palliative Care in the Metastatic Spinal Tumors. A Systematic Review on the Radiotherapy and Surgical Perspective. *Life* **2022**, *12*, 571. [CrossRef]
31. Fukushima, H.; Koga, F. Impact of sarcopenia in bladder preservation therapy for muscle-invasive bladder cancer patients: A narrative review. *Transl. Androl. Urol.* **2022**, *11*, 1433–1441. [CrossRef] [PubMed]
32. Tanaka, H.; Fukushima, H.; Kijima, T.; Nakamura, Y.; Yajima, S.; Uehara, S.; Yoshida, S.; Yokoyama, M.; Ishioka, J.; Matsuoka, Y.; et al. Feasibility and outcomes of selective tetramodal bladder-preservation therapy in elderly patients with muscle-invasive bladder cancer. *Int. J. Urol.* **2020**, *27*, 236–243. [CrossRef] [PubMed]
33. Iinuma, M.; Akazawa, T.; Torii, Y.; Ueno, J.; Yoshida, A.; Tomochika, K.; Hideshima, T.; Haraguchi, N.; Niki, H. Impact of nutritional status in patients with metastatic spinal tumors who underwent palliative surgery. *J. Orthop. Sci.* **2024**. [CrossRef] [PubMed]
34. Ramos, R.D.l.G.; Ryvlin, J.; Hamad, M.K.; Fourman, M.S.; Gelfand, Y.; Murthy, S.G.; Shin, J.H.; Yassari, R. Predictive value of six nutrition biomarkers in oncological spine surgery: A performance assessment for prediction of mortality and wound infection. *J. Neurosurgery: Spine* **2023**, *39*, 664–670. [CrossRef]

35. Tsantes, A.G.; Papadopoulos, D.V.; Lytras, T.; Tsantes, A.E.; Mavrogenis, A.F.; Koulouvaris, P.; Gelalis, I.D.; Ploumis, A.; Korompilias, A.V.; Benzakour, T.; et al. Association of malnutrition with surgical site infection following spinal surgery: Systematic review and meta-analysis. *J. Hosp. Infect.* **2020**, *104*, 111–119. [CrossRef]
36. Rigney, G.H.; Massaad, E.; Kiapour, A.; Razak, S.S.; Duvall, J.B.; Burrows, A.; Khalid, S.I.; Ramos, R.D.L.G.; Tobert, D.G.; Williamson, T.; et al. Implication of nutritional status for adverse outcomes after surgery for metastatic spine tumors. *J. Neurosurgery: Spine* **2023**, *39*, 557–567. [CrossRef]
37. Ferini, G.; Palmisciano, P.; Scalia, G.; Haider, A.S.; Bin-Alamer, O.; Sagoo, N.S.; Bozkurt, I.; Deora, H.; Priola, S.M.; Aoun, S.G.; et al. The role of radiation therapy in the treatment of spine metastases from hepatocellular carcinoma: A systematic review and meta-analysis. *Neurosurg. Focus* **2022**, *53*, E12. [CrossRef]

Journal of
Clinical Medicine

Article

Impact of the Spinal Instability Neoplastic Score on Postoperative Prognosis in Patients with Metastatic Cancer of the Cervical Spine

Dong-Ho Kang [1,†], Kyunghun Jung [1,†], Jin-Sung Park [1], Minwook Kang [1], Chong-Suh Lee [2] and Se-Jun Park [1,*]

1 Department of Orthopedic Surgery, Samsung Medical Center, Seoul 06351, Republic of Korea; ilucky7ik@gmail.com (K.J.); npng4eve@gmail.com (M.K.)
2 Department of Orthopedic Surgery, Haeundae Bumin Hospital, Busan 48094, Republic of Korea
* Correspondence: sejunos@gmail.com; Tel.: +82-2-3410-1583
† These authors contributed equally to this work.

Abstract: Background: Although the Spinal Instability Neoplastic Score (SINS) is widely utilized to evaluate spinal instability, its prognostic value for survival in patients with cervical spinal metastases remains unclear. This study investigated the association between the SINS and survival outcomes in patients with metastatic cervical spine cancer. **Methods:** This retrospective cohort study included 106 patients who underwent surgery for metastatic cervical spine cancer at a single institution between 1995 and 2023. Patients were divided into two groups: high SINS (≥13) and low-to-moderate SINS (0–12). Overall survival (OS) was the primary outcome and was analyzed using Kaplan–Meier estimates and Cox regression. Secondary outcomes included changes in Eastern Cooperative Oncology Group Performance Status (ECOG-PS), operation time, estimated blood loss, and postoperative complications. **Results:** The median OS was significantly shorter in the high SINS group compared to the low-to-moderate SINS group (5.3 months versus 8.6 months; $p = 0.023$). A high SINS was independently associated with increased mortality risk (hazard ratio [HR], 1.959; 95% CI, 1.221–3.143; $p = 0.005$). Lung cancer (HR, 4.004; 95% CI, 1.878–8.535; $p < 0.001$) and rectal cancer (HR, 3.293; 95% CI, 1.126–9.632; $p = 0.029$) were predictive of worse survival, whereas postoperative chemotherapy (HR, 0.591; 95% CI, 0.381–0.917; $p = 0.019$) and radiotherapy (HR, 0.531; 95% CI, 0.340–0.827; $p = 0.005$) were associated with improved survival. Changes in the ECOG-PS and postoperative complication rates were not significantly different between the groups. **Conclusions:** A high SINS was associated with significantly shorter survival in patients with metastatic cervical spine cancer, reflecting both mechanical instability and tumor aggressiveness.

Keywords: metastatic cancer of the cervical spine; Spinal Instability Neoplastic Score; overall survival; prognostic factors; surgical outcomes; spinal instability

1. Introduction

Metastatic cancer of the cervical spine is the third most common site of spinal metastasis after the thoracic and lumbar spine and presents unique challenges due to the distinct anatomical and biomechanical characteristics of the cervical spine [1–5]. The cervical spine's lack of rib support and high mobility increases its susceptibility to instability [6]. In this context, evaluating spinal stability in metastatic cancer of the cervical spine is crucial not only for preventing catastrophic events such as neurological compromise, but also for planning effective cervical-specific surgical and non-surgical treatments [7].

The Spinal Instability Neoplastic Score (SINS) has been widely used to assess the stability of spinal metastases [8]. This score was initially developed using the modified Delphi technique, focusing solely on spinal instability, and has therefore been traditionally regarded as unrelated to survival outcomes [9], with studies reporting no real associations [10–12]. For this reason, many prognostic scoring systems for spinal metastases exclude SINS [13–16]. However, a recent study suggested that a high SINS may be associated with poor prognosis [17], challenging the initial understanding of its prognostic value.

Although the prognostic value of the SINS remains controversial, its potential implications for metastatic cancer of the cervical spine remain unknown. The unique anatomy and biomechanics of the cervical spine affect both surgical approaches and outcomes, highlighting the need for focused studies on the prognostic value of the SINS. Therefore, this study sought to address this gap by examining the surgical outcomes in patients with high and low SINS. We compared surgical outcomes between high SINS groups ($\geq$13) and low-to-moderate SINS groups (0–12), evaluating whether SINS can serve as a meaningful predictor of prognosis and other treatment outcomes.

2. Materials and Methods

2.1. Study Design and Ethical Considerations

This retrospective cohort study was conducted at a single tertiary referral center specializing in spinal oncology. Data were obtained from the center's prospective Spinal Metastasis Registry. The study protocol was reviewed and approved by the Institutional Review Board (IRB) of Samsung Medical Center (IRB Approval Number: 2024-11-070). The requirement for informed consent was waived due to the retrospective nature of the study. Patient confidentiality was maintained by anonymizing the data and adhering to the principles outlined in the Declaration of Helsinki. Data were collected from electronic medical records and patient's picture archiving and communication systems.

2.2. Participants

Patients who underwent surgical treatment for metastatic cervical cancer at our institution between January 1995 and December 2023 were included in this retrospective cohort study. Eligible participants were identified using an institutional electronic medical records system. The inclusion criteria were as follows: (1) spinal metastasis diagnosed between 1995 and 2023 and (2) surgical treatment specifically for cervical spinal metastasis. The exclusion criteria were as follows: (1) incomplete or inaccurate clinical and radiological data necessary for SINS evaluation and (2) death due to non-tumor-related causes. The patients were categorized into two groups based on their SINS: high and low-to-moderate.

2.3. Outcome Measures and Data Collection

The primary outcome was overall survival (OS), which was defined as the time from surgery to death from any cause, with surviving patients censored at the last follow-up. Secondary outcomes included postoperative changes in the Eastern Cooperative Oncology Group-Performance Status (ECOG-PS), surgical burden including operation time, estimated blood loss, postoperative complications, and independent predictors of survival identified through Cox regression analysis.

Patient demographic and baseline characteristics, including age, sex, primary cancer type, ECOG-PS, Frankel grade, and Karnofsky Performance Status (KPS), were retrospectively extracted. Tumor-specific variables, such as SINS, number of extraspinal bony metastases, visceral metastases, and primary location of cervical lesions, were recorded along with preoperative and postoperative therapeutic interventions, including chemotherapy and radiotherapy.

Surgical variables documented included operation type (e.g., anterior debulking and fixation, posterior debulking and fixation, and fixation), operation time, and estimated blood loss. Anterior debulking and fixation included procedures performed using either an anterior only or combined anterior and posterior approach. Complications, including wound infections, fractures, and tumor relapse-associated neurological deterioration, were recorded. Postoperative functional changes were assessed by comparing preoperative and postoperative ECOG-PS scores and categorizing the patients into improved, unchanged, or aggravated groups.

2.4. Statistical Analysis

Continuous variables are expressed as means with standard deviations or medians with interquartile ranges, as appropriate. Categorical variables are presented as frequencies and percentages. Comparisons between the high and low-to-moderate SINS groups were conducted using the independent two-sample t-test or Mann–Whitney U test for continuous variables and the chi-square test or Fisher's exact test for categorical variables. Survival outcomes were analyzed using Kaplan–Meier survival estimates, and the log-rank test was used to compare survival distributions between the groups. Median OS was reported with a 95% confidence interval (CI). Univariate and multivariate Cox proportional hazards regression analyses were conducted to identify independent predictors of survival. Variables with p-values < 0.10 in univariate analysis were included in the multivariate model. Hazard ratios (HRs) with 95% CIs were calculated to quantify the strength of the association. Postoperative changes in ECOG-PS were analyzed using paired comparisons of pre- and postoperative scores within each group using chi-squared analysis. Statistical analyses were performed using SPSS (version 27.0; SPSS Inc., Chicago, IL, USA), and statistical significance was set at $p < 0.05$.

3. Results

3.1. Participant Characteristics and Comparison of Low-to-Moderate and High SINS Groups

Ultimately, 106 patients who underwent surgical treatment for metastatic cervical cancer between January 1995 and December 2023 were included in this study. A total of 71 patients (67.0%) were allocated to the low-to-moderate SINS group and 35 (33.0%) to the high SINS group. The baseline characteristics of the patients are summarized in Table 1. The mean age of all participants was 58.2 ± 10.1 years. Male patients comprised 57.5% of the cohort. Lung cancer (26.4%) and liver cancer (19.8%) were the most common primary tumor types, followed by breast cancer (12.3%), colorectal cancer (5.7%), and kidney cancer (4.7%). There were no significant differences between the two groups in terms of age, sex, or primary tumor type. Furthermore, measures of functional and performance statuses, including ECOG-PS, Frankel grade, and KPS, were comparable between the groups. Other characteristics, such as the number of vertebral body metastases, presence of visceral metastases, number of extraspinal bony metastases, and perioperative chemotherapy and radiotherapy, also showed no significant differences. Similarly, the main locations of the cervical lesions were evenly distributed between the groups. Significant differences were observed between surgical approaches. Surgical strategies differed between the groups, with patients with high SINS undergoing anterior debulking more frequently than those with low to moderate SINS; however, the difference was not significant (71.4% vs. 49.3%; $p = 0.105$).

Table 1. Baseline characteristics of all patients and their comparison across the low-to-moderate and high SINS groups.

Characteristics	All Patients (N = 106)	Low-to-Moderate SINS (N = 71)	High SINS (N = 35)	p-Value
Age, year, mean ± SD	58.2 ± 10.1	58.9 ± 9.7	56.8 ± 10.9	0.321
Male, n (%)	61 (57.5)	44 (62.0)	17 (48.6)	0.189
Primary cancer, n (%)				
Lung	28 (26.4)	21 (29.6)	7 (20.0)	
Liver	21 (19.8)	17 (23.9)	4 (11.4)	
Breast	13 (12.3)	6 (8.5)	7 (20.0)	
Colorectal	6 (5.7)	5 (7.0)	1 (2.9)	0.086
Kidney	5 (4.7)	4 (5.6)	1 (2.9)	
Prostate	2 (1.9)	2 (2.8)	0 (0.0)	
Thyroid	2 (1.9)	2 (2.8)	0 (0.0)	
Others	29 (27.4)	14 (19.7)	15 (42.9)	

Table 1. *Cont.*

Characteristics	All Patients (N = 106)	Low-to-Moderate SINS (N = 71)	High SINS (N = 35)	*p*-Value
ECOG-PS, n (%)				
0	2 (1.9)	1 (1.4)	1 (2.9)	0.559
1	40 (37.7)	30 (42.3)	10 (28.6)	
2	35 (33.0)	22 (31.0)	13 (37.1)	
3	23 (21.7)	15 (21.1)	8 (22.9)	
4	6 (5.7)	3 (4.2)	3 (8.6)	
Frankel grade, n (%)				
E	48 (45.3)	32 (45.1)	16 (45.7)	0.999
C and D	56 (52.8)	37 (52.1)	19 (54.3)	
A and B	2 (1.9)	2 (2.8)	0 (0.0)	
Karnofsky performance status, n (%)				
Good (80–100%)	34 (32.1)	24 (33.8)	10 (28.6)	0.841
Moderate (50–70%)	53 (50.0)	35 (49.3)	18 (51.4)	
Poor (10–40%)	19 (17.9)	12 (16.9)	7 (20.0)	
Number of extraspinal bony metastases, n (%)				
0	50 (47.2)	31 (43.7)	19 (54.3)	0.572
1–2	23 (21.7)	17 (23.9)	6 (17.1)	
≥3	33 (31.1)	23 (32.4)	10 (28.6)	
Metastasis to visceral organs, n (%)				
No metastases	56 (52.8)	38 (53.5)	18 (51.4)	0.999
Removable	5 (4.7)	3 (4.2)	2 (5.7)	
Unremovable	45 (42.5)	30 (42.3)	15 (42.9)	
Number of metastases in the vertebral body, n (%)				
1	32 (30.2)	22 (31.0)	10 (28.6)	0.345
2	26 (24.5)	20 (28.2)	6 (17.1)	
≥3	48 (45.3)	29 (40.8)	19 (54.3)	
Main cervical lesion				
C1	1 (0.9)	1 (1.4)	0 (0.0)	0.482
C2	18 (17.0)	15 (21.1)	3 (8.6)	
C3	9 (8.5)	7 (9.9)	2 (5.7)	
C4	20 (18.9)	12 (16.9)	8 (22.9)	
C5	15 (14.2)	10 (14.1)	5 (14.3)	
C6	21 (19.8)	11 (15.5)	10 (28.6)	
C7	22 (20.8)	15 (21.1)	7 (20.0)	
SINS				
0–6	7 (6.6)	7 (9.9)	0 (0.0)	<0.001
7–12	64 (60.4)	64 (90.1)	0 (0.0)	
≥13	35 (33.0)	0 (0.0)	35 (100.0)	
Operation type, n (%)				
Fixation only	15 (14.2)	12 (16.9)	3 (8.6)	0.105
Posterior debulking and fixation	31 (29.2)	24 (33.8)	7 (20.0)	
Anterior debulking and fixation	60 (56.6)	35 (49.3)	25 (71.4)	
Usage of occiput plate	8 (7.5)	6 (8.5)	2 (5.7)	0.999
Preoperative chemotherapy, n (%)	56 (52.8)	36 (50.7)	20 (57.1)	0.532
Preoperative radiotherapy, n (%)	38 (26.4)	24 (33.8)	14 (40.0)	0.532
Postoperative chemotherapy, n (%)	50 (47.2)	33 (46.5)	17 (48.6)	0.839
Postoperative radiotherapy, n (%)	64 (60.4)	45 (63.4)	19 (54.3)	0.368

3.2. Survival Analysis

The median estimated survival for all patients was 7.1 months (95% CI, 5.3–8.9) (Figure 1). Kaplan–Meier survival analysis demonstrated a significantly shorter median survival in the high SINS group (5.3 months; 95% CI, 3.8–6.8) compared to the low-to-moderate SINS group (8.6 months; 95% CI, 6.9–10.2; $p = 0.023$) (Figure 2).

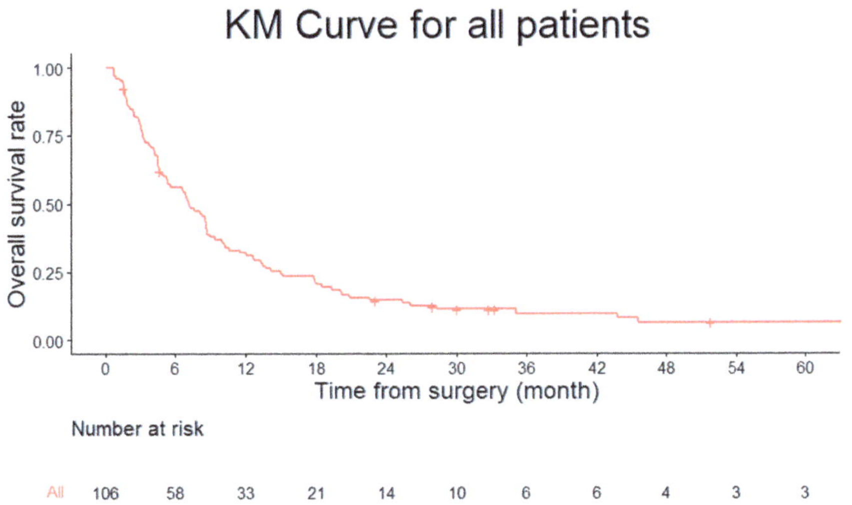

Figure 1. Kaplan–Meier survival curve showing the overall survival of 106 patients with metastatic cervical spine cancer.

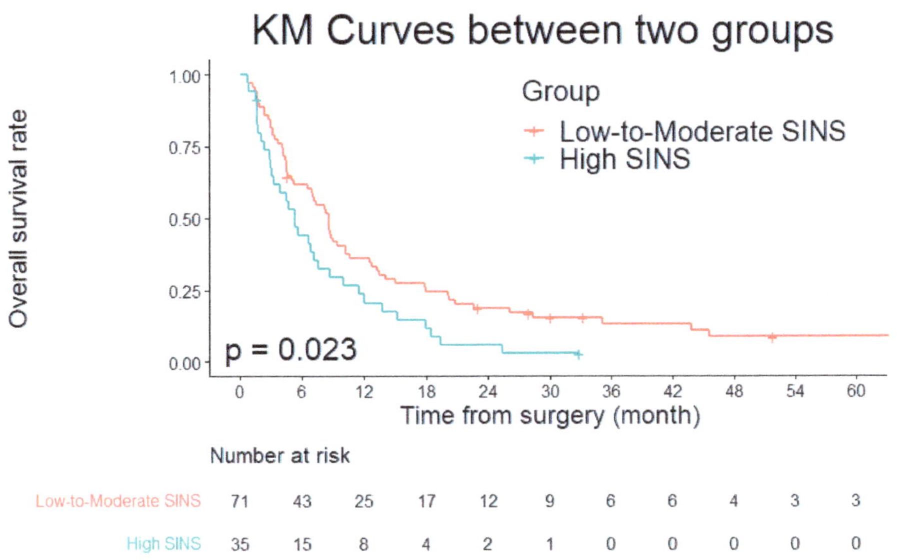

Figure 2. Kaplan–Meier survival curve comparing overall survival between the low-to-moderate SINS group (median survival: 8.6 months) and the high SINS group (median survival: 5.3 months; $p = 0.023$).

3.3. Changes in Functional Status

In the low-to-moderate SINS group, 18.3% of patients revealed improvements in ECOG-PS, 53.5% showed no change, and 26.8% experienced worsening of their performance status (Table 2). Similarly, in the high SINS group, 17.1% of the patients demonstrated improvement, 54.3% showed no change, and 28.6% had worsening ECOG-PS (Table 3). There was no significant difference between the two groups in the proportion of patients with improved ECOG-PS after surgery (p = 0.883) or those with worsening ECOG-PS (p = 0.844).

Table 2. The number of patients showing postoperative changes in ECOG-PS after surgery in the low-to-moderate SINS group.

Preoperative ECOG-PS	Postoperative ECOG-PS						Total
	0	**1**	**2**	**3**	**4**	**5**	
0	0	1 [b]	0 [b]	0 [b]	0 [b]	0 [b]	1
1	1 [a]	17	7 [b]	3 [b]	1 [b]	1 [b]	30
2	0 [a]	2 [a]	15	5 [b]	0 [b]	0 [b]	22
3	0 [a]	1 [a]	6 [a]	7	1 [b]	0 [b]	15
4	0 [a]	0 [a]	1 [a]	2 [a]	0	0 [b]	3
Total	1	21	29	17	2	1	71

Light grey box [a]: improved ECOG-PS; white box: no change in ECOG-PS; dark grey box [b]: aggravated ECOG-PS; SINS, Spinal Instability Neoplastic Scale; ECOG-PS, Eastern Cooperative Oncology Group-Performance Status.

Table 3. The number of patients demonstrating postoperative changes in ECOG-PS after surgery in the high SINS group.

Preoperative ECOG-PS	Postoperative ECOG-PS						Total
	0	**1**	**2**	**3**	**4**	**5**	
0	1	0 [b]	0 [b]	0 [b]	0 [b]	0 [b]	1
1	0 [a]	5	4 [b]	1 [b]	0 [b]	0 [b]	10
2	0 [a]	1 [a]	9	2 [b]	1 [b]	0 [b]	13
3	0 [a]	0 [a]	4 [a]	3	1 [b]	0 [b]	8
4	0 [a]	0 [a]	0 [a]	1 [a]	1	1 [b]	3
Total	1	6	17	7	3	1	35

Light grey box [a]: improved ECOG-PS; white box: no change in ECOG-PS; dark grey box [b]: aggravated ECOG-PS; SINS, Spinal Instability Neoplastic Scale; ECOG-PS, Eastern Cooperative Oncology Group-Performance Status.

3.4. Surgical Burden and Postoperative Complications

The mean operation time for all patients was 5.6 ± 2.2 h, with the low-to-moderate SINS group having a longer mean operation time compared to the high SINS group (5.9 ± 2.5 h vs. 5.0 ± 1.5 h; p = 0.020) (Table 4). However, there was no significant difference in the estimated blood loss between the two groups (low-to-moderate SINS: 684.5 ± 1215.9 mL vs. high SINS: 553.4 ± 473.4 mL; p = 0.541). Postoperative complications were comparable between the groups (Figure 3). The overall rate of revision surgeries due to complications was low in both groups, with four patients (5.6%) in the low-to-moderate SINS group and three patients (8.6%) in the high SINS group requiring additional interventions (p = 0.682). The overall rate of wound infection was 3.8%, with no significant difference between the groups (p = 0.597). In the low-to-moderate SINS group, two patients (2.8%) experienced wound infections compared to two patients (5.7%) in the high SINS group. Further fractures were rare, occurring in only one patient (2.9%) in the high SINS group, whereas no cases were reported in the low-to-moderate SINS group (p = 0.330). Tumor relapse-associated neurological deterioration was noted in two patients (2.8%) in the low-to-moderate SINS group, whereas no cases occurred in the high SINS group (p = 0.999).

Table 4. Surgical burden and perioperative complications of all patients and their comparison across the low-to-moderate and high SINS groups.

	All Patients (N = 106)	Low-to-Moderate SINS (N = 71)	High SINS (N = 35)	p-Value
Surgical variables				
Operation time (h)	5.6 ± 2.2	5.9 ± 2.5	5.0 ± 1.5	0.020
Estimated blood loss (mL)	641.2 ± 1030.5	684.5 ± 1215.9	553.4 ± 473.4	0.541
Surgical complications				
Total events requiring revision surgery, n (%)	7 (6.6)	4 (5.6)	3 (8.6)	0.682
Wound infection, n (%)	4 (3.8)	2 (2.8)	2 (5.7)	0.597
Increased neurology due to tumor relapse, n (%)	2 (1.9)	2 (2.8)	0 (0.0)	0.999
Further fracture, n (%)	1 (0.9)	0 (0.0)	1 (2.9)	0.330

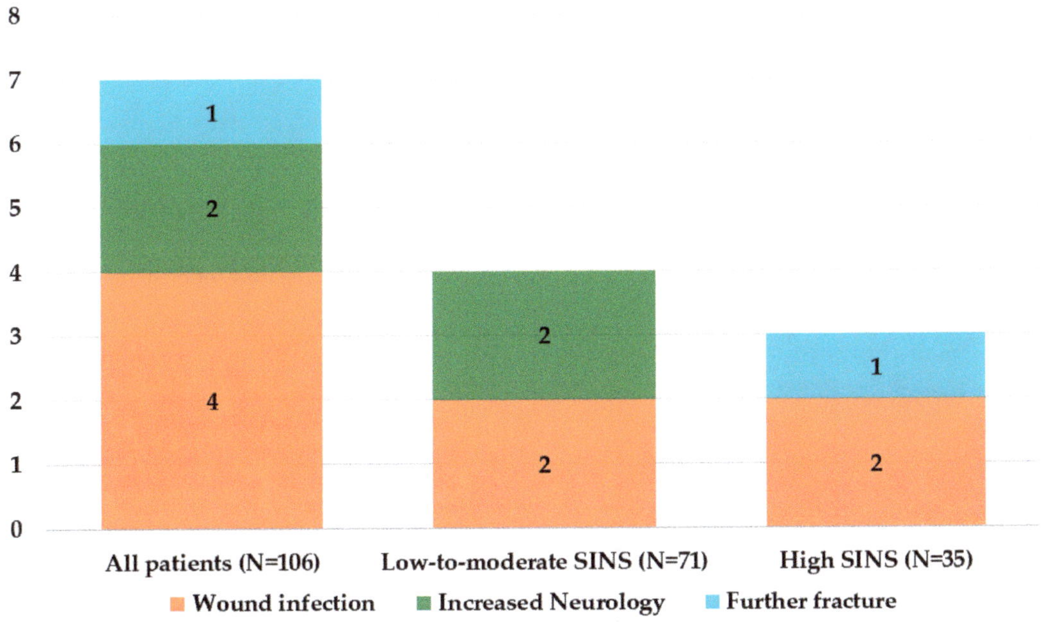

Figure 3. Surgical complications across the low-to-moderate and high SINS groups.

3.5. Cox Regression Analysis

In the multivariate analysis, a high SINS was identified as an independent predictor of increased mortality risk (HR, 1.959; 95% CI, 1.221–3.143; $p = 0.005$) (Table 5). Specific primary tumor origins included lung cancer (hazard ratio [HR], 4.004; 95% [CI], 1.878–8.535; $p < 0.001$) and rectal cancer (HR, 3.293; 95% CI, 1.126–9.632; $p = 0.029$). Conversely, postoperative chemotherapy (HR, 0.591; 95% CI, 0.381–0.917; $p = 0.019$) and radiotherapy (HR, 0.531; 95% CI, 0.340–0.827; $p = 0.005$) were independently associated with a reduced mortality risk.

Table 5. Cox regression analysis identifying factors associated with mortality.

	Univariate Analysis		Multivariate Analysis	
	Hazard Ratio (95% CI)	*p* Value	Hazard Ratio (95% CI)	*p* Value
Sex (male)		0.086		0.430
Low-to-moderate SINS	Reference			
High SINS	1.637 (1.064–2.517)	0.025	1.959 (1.221–3.143)	0.005
Preoperative Frankel grade	0.639 (0.429–0.950)	0.026		0.084
Modified Tokuhashi score	0.923 (0.847–1.006)	0.067		0.838
Primary cancer group of the modified Tokuhashi score		0.003		0.008
5 (thyroid, breast, prostate, carcinoid tumor)	Reference			
4 (rectum)	3.049 (1.099–8.459)	0.032	3.293 (1.126–9.632)	0.029
3 (kidney, uterus)	1.314 (0.417–4.138)	0.641		0.337
2 (other)	3.154 (1.556–6.394)	0.001	2.648 (1.295–5.415)	0.008
1 (liver, gallbladder)	2.636 (1.240–5.605)	0.012	2.715 (1.227–6.011)	0.014
0 (lung, pancreas, etc.)	3.686 (1.777–7.646)	<0.001	4.004 (1.878–8.535)	<0.001
Preoperative radiotherapy	1.866 (1.217–2.860)	0.004		0.881
Postoperative chemotherapy	0.477 (0.314–0.725)	0.001	0.591 (0.381–0.917)	0.019
Postoperative radiotherapy	0.502 (0.330–0.763)	0.001	0.531 (0.340–0.827)	0.005

4. Discussion

This study highlights the prognostic significance of the SINS in patients with metastatic cervical spine cancer. Our findings show that a high SINS is independently associated with reduced overall survival, with patients in this group exhibiting a median survival of only 5.3 months compared with 8.6 months in the low-to-moderate SINS group. Conversely, postoperative chemotherapy and radiotherapy were shown to improve survival.

SINS was initially developed to predict spinal instability requiring surgical fixation rather than patient survival. Our findings suggest that SINS may have additional prognostic value in patients with metastatic cervical spine cancer due to its unique biomechanical considerations. In the literature, the relationship between SINS and survival outcomes has been debated. Previous studies have reported conflicting results regarding the prognostic value [10–12,17]. Ha et al. reported no direct impact of SINS on survival in metastatic lung and hepatocellular cancers, emphasizing the importance of performance status and systemic treatment [10]. Zadnik et al. found no significant association between SINS and survival in patients undergoing surgery for multiple myeloma, indicating that SINS primarily reflects mechanical instability rather than tumor aggressiveness [12]. However, their study reported that the mean SINS was higher in patients who survived more than 1 year compared to those who survived less than 1 year (11 $\pm$ 2.6 months vs. 8.5 $\pm$ 2.4 months; $p = 0.056$). They also showed that the Kaplan–Meier survival curves for indeterminate stability (SINS 7–12) and instability (SINS 13–18) were clearly separated. However, the difference in survival between the two groups was not statistically significant based on the log-rank test ($p = 0.12$). Although the difference was not statistically significant, this may be attributed to the small sample size (31 patients). Another study by Zadnik assessed an observational cohort of 43 patients who underwent surgical resection for metastatic breast cancer and investigated the impact of SINS [11]. In this analysis, there was no statistically significant difference in survival between patients with SINSs indicating indeterminate stability (7–12) versus gross instability (13–18). However, the median survival was only 12.7 months in the unstable group compared to 28.1 months for the indeterminately stable groups, respectively. The groups were similar in terms of the surgical level, preoperative KPS, and patient age. Importantly, the SINS data were based on 22 patients, and the lack of statistical significance may be attributable to the small sample size.

However, recent studies have challenged these findings. Versteeg et al. reviewed the use of the SINS in clinical practice and identified studies suggesting a potential link between higher SINSs and poorer outcomes, particularly in patients with high systemic tumor burdens [9]. Similarly, Miyaji et al. evaluated the SINS in castration-resistant prostate cancer and revealed that patients with unstable spines (SINS $\geq$ 7) had a significantly reduced survival compared to those with stable spines (SINS $\leq$ 6), with a hazard ratio of 2.60 (95% CI, 1.07–5.93; p = 0.0345), which is echoed by our result [17]. A possible explanation for these results is the hypothesis that high SINSs may not only signify mechanical instability but also reflect the biological aggressiveness of the tumor and a higher predisposition for systemic spread. Patients with high SINSs in our cohort exhibited a significantly shorter median survival (5.3 months) compared to those with low-to-moderate scores (8.6 months), reinforcing the prognostic relevance of this tool in this specific patient population. This finding underscores the dual role of the SINS as both a stability assessment tool and an indicator of tumor severity, particularly in the context of cervical spine metastases. Cervical lesions are more prone to instability than thoracic lesions, which are supported by ribs. As a result, the onset of symptoms prompting surgery is likely to be similar between the low and high SINS groups. Therefore, a higher SINS, which reflects greater bone destruction at the time of surgery, may indicate more aggressive tumor characteristics. The SINS may also serve as a complementary tool in prognostic evaluations for patients with metastatic cervical spine cancer. A high SINS can suggest a prognosis that is potentially worse than what previous legacy prognostic models predicted. This should be taken into account when assessing the suitability of surgical intervention and in choosing the appropriate surgical method. Furthermore, surgeons and oncologists could consider integrating the SINS into existing prognostic systems or utilizing it to develop new scoring models tailored specifically to cervical spine metastases.

Interestingly, the proportion of patients with unchanged ECOG-PS was higher than that of patients with improvement or worsening, indicating that while surgery may stabilize functional status, achieving substantial recovery is challenging. Specifically, 28.6% of patients in the high SINS group and 26.8% in the low-to-moderate SINS group had deteriorated ECOG-PS, whereas only 17.1% and 18.3%, respectively, demonstrated improvement. This aligns with the findings of Moon et al., who observed that spinal decompression surgery often prevents further neurological decline but does not guarantee significant functional improvement, particularly in advanced cancer [18].

In Table 4, the operation time was slightly longer in the low-to-moderate SINS group (p = 0.020). This difference may be attributed to the relatively higher proportion of C2 lesions in the low-to-moderate SINS group, as C2 lesions typically require more complex surgical approaches. However, from a clinical perspective, this difference in operation time is not considered to be of significant importance, as it did not influence other perioperative outcomes or overall survival. Estimated blood loss and perioperative complication rates were comparable between the two groups, except for operation time. This similarity likely reflects that the choice of surgical approach in cervical lesions is typically determined by the tumor's location (anterior or posterior) rather than the SINS. As a result, both groups underwent similar surgical procedures, which may explain the lack of significant differences in surgical burden and perioperative complications. In our study, the total adverse event rate was 8.5%, which was notably lower than the rates reported in other studies on surgical interventions for spinal metastases. Lau et al. reported an overall complication rate of 21.7% in a cohort of patients undergoing surgery for spinal metastasis [19]. Tan et al. also reported a 20.7% surgical complication rate in patients who underwent surgery for spinal metastases [20]. This disparity can be explained by the influence of the survival duration on the reported incidence of postoperative complications. In a study by Tan et al., the median survival of all patients was 16 months, allowing a longer window for the development of postoperative complications. Conversely, the median survival in our cohort was only 7.1 months, which was significantly shorter and likely limited the time frame for adverse events to occur. Further research is required to clarify whether patients with metastatic cervical cancer have inferior survival rates after surgical treatment.

This study has several limitations. First, its retrospective design inherently introduced a selection bias, as only patients who underwent surgical treatment were included. This may limit the generalizability of the findings to patients managed with nonsurgical treatments or those with less severe disease. Second, the study was conducted at a single tertiary referral center, which may have restricted the applicability of the results to other institutions with different patient populations and management practices. Third, the relatively small sample size, particularly in the high SINS group, may have limited the statistical power to detect subtle differences in secondary outcomes such as functional status changes and complication rates. Fourth, there is a possibility of survivor bias. As only patients who underwent surgery were included, those with more severe conditions who were ineligible for surgery may be underrepresented. This could have influenced survival and outcome findings. Fifth, there is no consideration of benign aggressive tumors, such as giant cell tumors, which can also cause instability. For giant cell tumors, aggressive surgical interventions and denosumab therapy are essential for achieving favorable outcomes [21]. Future studies should include these types of tumors. Furthermore, the use of historical data spanning nearly three decades (1995–2023) introduces potential variability in surgical techniques, perioperative care, and adjunctive therapies that may influence patient outcomes. For instance, the introduction of targeted chemotherapy has revolutionized the treatment landscape for metastatic cancer, offering more effective systemic control and potentially influencing survival outcomes. While stratified analysis by decade or surgical technique could provide valuable insights, the limited sample size in each decade would likely result in insufficient statistical power for meaningful results. Therefore, future prospective studies should aim to validate these findings in larger multicenter cohorts to reduce bias and enhance the reliability of the results.

5. Conclusions

This study demonstrated that high SINSs ($\geq$13) in patients with metastatic cervical spine cancer were associated with poorer survival outcomes. In these patients, SINS can serve as a dual-purpose tool, highlighting mechanical instability and providing insights into the biological behavior of the tumor. Patients with high SINSs had a significantly shorter median survival (5.3 months) than those in the low-to-moderate SINS group (8.6 months). These findings support the integration of the SINS into patient management strategies, either as a complementary tool for prognostic evaluations or as part of novel scoring systems, to improve prognostic accuracy and guide treatment decisions. Future studies should aim to validate these findings in larger, multicenter cohorts and explore the integration of SINS into comprehensive prognostic models.

Author Contributions: Conceptualization, D.-H.K. and S.-J.P.; methodology, D.-H.K. and S.-J.P.; software, D.-H.K. and K.J.; validation, D.-H.K. and K.J.; formal analysis, D.-H.K. and K.J.; resources, D.-H.K. and K.J.; data curation, K.J. and M.K.; writing—original draft preparation, D.-H.K.; writing—review and editing, D.-H.K. and S.-J.P.; visualization, D.-H.K.; supervision, J.-S.P., C.-S.L. and S.-J.P.; project administration, J.-S.P., C.-S.L. and S.-J.P. All authors have read and agreed to the published version of the manuscript.

Funding: This study received no external funding.

Institutional Review Board Statement: This study was conducted in accordance with the Declaration of Helsinki. The study protocol was approved by the Institutional Review Board of Samsung Medical Center (IRB number: 2024-11-070; Date: 18 November 2024).

Informed Consent Statement: Informed consent was obtained from all the participants involved in the study.

Data Availability Statement: Data underlying this article cannot be shared publicly because of the privacy of individuals who participated in the study. The data can be shared by the corresponding authors upon reasonable request.

Conflicts of Interest: The authors declare no conflict of interest. The funders had no role in the study design, collection, analyses, interpretation of data, writing of the manuscript, or decision to publish the results.

References

1. Sciubba, D.M.; Petteys, R.J.; Dekutoski, M.B.; Fisher, C.G.; Fehlings, M.G.; Ondra, S.L.; Rhines, L.D.; Gokaslan, Z.L. Diagnosis and management of metastatic spine disease: A review. *J. Neurosurg. Spine* **2010**, *13*, 94–108. [CrossRef] [PubMed]
2. Hong, S.H.; Chang, B.-S.; Kim, H.; Kang, D.-H.; Chang, S.Y. An Updated Review on the Treatment Strategy for Spinal Metastasis from the Spine Surgeon's Perspective. *Asian Spine J.* **2022**, *16*, 799–811. [CrossRef] [PubMed]
3. Chang, S.Y.; Mok, S.; Park, S.C.; Kim, H.; Chang, B.S. Treatment Strategy for Metastatic Spinal Tumors: A Narrative Review. *Asian Spine J.* **2020**, *14*, 513–525. [CrossRef] [PubMed]
4. Park, S.J.; Park, J.S.; Lee, C.S.; Kang, B.J.; Jung, C.W. Trends in Survival and Surgical Methods in Patients Surgically Treated for Metastatic Spinal Tumors: 25-Year Experience in a Single Institution. *Clin. Orthop. Surg.* **2023**, *15*, 109–117. [CrossRef]
5. Kim, Y.H.; Kim, J.; Chang, S.Y.; Kim, H.; Chang, B.S. Treatment Strategy for Impending Instability in Spinal Metastases. *Clin. Orthop. Surg.* **2020**, *12*, 337–342. [CrossRef]
6. Bogduk, N.; Mercer, S. Biomechanics of the cervical spine. I: Normal kinematics. *Clin. Biomech.* **2000**, *15*, 633–648. [CrossRef]
7. Molina, C.A.; Gokaslan, Z.L.; Sciubba, D.M. Diagnosis and management of metastatic cervical spine tumors. *Orthop. Clin. N. Am.* **2012**, *43*, 75–87. [CrossRef]
8. Fisher, C.G.; Dipaola, C.P.; Ryken, T.C.; Bilsky, M.H.; Shaffrey, C.I.; Berven, S.H.; Harrop, J.S.; Fehlings, M.G.; Boriani, S.; Chou, D.; et al. A novel classification system for spinal instability in neoplastic disease: An evidence-based approach and expert consensus from the spine oncology study group. *Spine* **2010**, *35*, E1221–E1229. [CrossRef]
9. Versteeg, A.L.; Verlaan, J.J.; Sahgal, A.; Mendel, E.; Quraishi, N.A.; Fourney, D.R.; Fisher, C.G. The Spinal Instability Neoplastic Score: Impact on Oncologic Decision-Making. *Spine* **2016**, *41* (Suppl. S20), S231–S237. [CrossRef]
10. Ha, K.Y.; Kim, Y.H.; Ahn, J.H.; Park, H.Y. Factors Affecting Survival in Patients Undergoing Palliative Spine Surgery for Metastatic Lung and Hepatocellular Cancer: Dose the Type of Surgery Influence the Surgical Results for Metastatic Spine Disease? *Clin. Orthop. Surg.* **2015**, *7*, 344–350. [CrossRef]
11. Zadnik, P.L.; Hwang, L.; Ju, D.G.; Groves, M.L.; Sui, J.; Yurter, A.; Witham, T.F.; Bydon, A.; Wolinsky, J.P.; Gokaslan, Z.L.; et al. Prolonged survival following aggressive treatment for metastatic breast cancer in the spine. *Clin. Exp. Metastasis* **2014**, *31*, 47–55. [CrossRef] [PubMed]
12. Zadnik, P.L.; Goodwin, C.R.; Karami, K.J.; Mehta, A.I.; Amin, A.G.; Groves, M.L.; Wolinsky, J.P.; Witham, T.F.; Bydon, A.; Gokaslan, Z.L.; et al. Outcomes following surgical intervention for impending and gross instability caused by multiple myeloma in the spinal column. *J. Neurosurg. Spine* **2015**, *22*, 301–309. [CrossRef] [PubMed]
13. Tokuhashi, Y.; Matsuzaki, H.; Oda, H.; Oshima, M.; Ryu, J. A revised scoring system for preoperative evaluation of metastatic spine tumor prognosis. *Spine* **2005**, *30*, 2186–2191. [CrossRef] [PubMed]
14. Schoenfeld, A.J.; Ferrone, M.L.; Blucher, J.A.; Agaronnik, N.; Nguyen, L.; Tobert, D.G.; Balboni, T.A.; Schwab, J.H.; Shin, J.H.; Sciubba, D.M.; et al. Prospective comparison of the accuracy of the New England Spinal Metastasis Score (NESMS) to legacy scoring systems in prognosticating outcomes following treatment of spinal metastases. *Spine J.* **2022**, *22*, 39–48. [CrossRef]
15. Paulino Pereira, N.R.; Janssen, S.J.; van Dijk, E.; Harris, M.B.; Hornicek, F.J.; Ferrone, M.L.; Schwab, J.H. Development of a Prognostic Survival Algorithm for Patients with Metastatic Spine Disease. *J. Bone Jt. Surgery. Am. Vol.* **2016**, *98*, 1767–1776. [CrossRef]
16. Truong, V.T.; Al-Shakfa, F.; Roberge, D.; Masucci, G.L.; Tran, T.P.Y.; Dib, R.; Yuh, S.J.; Wang, Z. Assessing the Performance of Prognostic Scores in Patients with Spinal Metastases from Lung Cancer Undergoing Non-surgical Treatment. *Asian Spine J.* **2023**, *17*, 739–749. [CrossRef]
17. Miyaji, Y.; Nakanishi, K.; Yamamoto, A.; Yoden, E.; Tokiya, R.; Okawaki, M.; Inubushi, M.; Katsui, K. Spinal Instability as a Prognostic Factor in Patients with Spinal Metastasis of Castration-resistant Prostate Cancer. *Cancer Diagn. Progn.* **2023**, *3*, 449–456. [CrossRef]
18. Moon, K.Y.; Chung, C.K.; Jahng, T.A.; Kim, H.J.; Kim, C.H. Postoperative Survival and Ambulatory Outcome in Metastatic Spinal Tumors: Prognostic Factor Analysis. *J. Korean Neurosurg. Soc.* **2011**, *50*, 216–223. [CrossRef]
19. Lau, D.; Leach, M.R.; Than, K.D.; Ziewacz, J.; La Marca, F.; Park, P. Independent predictors of complication following surgery for spinal metastasis. *Eur. Spine J.* **2013**, *22*, 1402–1407. [CrossRef]

20. Tan, J.H.J.; Hallinan, J.; Ang, S.W.; Tan, T.H.; Tan, H.I.J.; Tan, L.T.I.; Sin, Q.S.; Lee, R.; Hey, H.W.D.; Chan, Y.H.; et al. Outcomes and Complications of Surgery for Symptomatic Spinal Metastases; a Comparison Between Patients Aged $\geq$ 70 and <70. *Glob. Spine J.* **2023**, 21925682231209624. [CrossRef]
21. Hashimoto, K.; Nishimura, S.; Miyamoto, H.; Toriumi, K.; Ikeda, T.; Akagi, M. Comprehensive treatment outcomes of giant cell tumor of the spine: A retrospective study. *Medicine* **2022**, *101*, e29963. [CrossRef]

Journal of
Clinical Medicine

MDPI

Article

Can Preoperative Hounsfield Unit Measurement Help Predict Mechanical Failure in Metastatic Spinal Tumor Surgery?

Hyung Rae Lee [1], Jae Hwan Cho [2,*], Sang Yun Seok [3], San Kim [2], Dae Wi Cho [2] and Jae Hyuk Yang [1]

1 Department of Orthopedic Surgery, Korea University Medical Center, Anam Hospital, Seoul 02841, Republic of Korea; drhrleeos@gmail.com (H.R.L.); kuspine@korea.ac.kr (J.H.Y.)
2 Department of Orthopedic Surgery, Asan Medical Center, University of Ulsan College of Medicine, Seoul 05505, Republic of Korea; kimrlatks2@naver.com (S.K.); zozo5313@gmail.com (D.W.C.)
3 Department of Orthopedic Surgery, Daejeon Eulji Medical Center, University of Eulji College of Medicine, Daejeon 35233, Republic of Korea; oper251@hanmail.net
* Correspondence: spinecjh@gmail.com; Tel.: +82-2-3010-3549; Fax: +82-2-3010-8555

Abstract: Background/Objectives: This study aimed to identify risk factors associated with mechanical failure in patients undergoing spinal instrumentation without fusion for metastatic spinal tumors. **Methods:** We retrospectively evaluated data from 220 patients with spinal tumors who underwent instrumentation without fusion. Propensity scores were used to match preoperative variables, resulting in the inclusion of 24 patients in the failure group (F group) and 72 in the non-failure group (non-F group). Demographic, surgical, and radiological characteristics were compared between the two groups. Logistic regression and Kaplan–Meier survival analyses were conducted to identify predictors of mechanical failure. **Results:** Propensity score matching resulted in a balanced distribution of covariates. Lower Hounsfield unit (HU) values at the lowest instrumented vertebra (LIV) were the only independent predictor of implant failure ($p = 0.037$). A cutoff value of 127.273 HUs was determined to predict mechanical failure, with a sensitivity of 59.1%, specificity of 73.4%, and area under the curve of 0.655 (95% confidence interval: 0.49–0.79). A significant difference in survival was observed between the groups with HU values above and below the cutoff ($p = 0.0057$). Cement-augmented screws were underutilized, with an average of only 0.2 screws per patient in the F group. **Conclusions:** Preoperative LIV HU values < 127.273 were strongly associated with an increased risk of mechanical failure following spinal instrumentation without fusion. Alternative surgical strategies including the use of cement-augmented screws are recommended for patients with low HU values.

Keywords: metastatic spinal tumors; instrumentation without fusion; Hounsfield units; mechanical failure; cement-augmented screws; propensity score matching

1. Introduction

Spinal metastatic tumors arise from various primary cancers and often cause pain, neurological symptoms, and spinal instability [1–3]. Surgical intervention is essential, particularly in cases of cord compression that promote neurological deficits or instability caused by metastasis [1,4]. Common surgical approaches include decompression or corpectomy with fixation, as well as en bloc excision and fixation. In many cases, fusion is not performed, and fixation alone is often preferred [1,4–6].

Achieving stable arthrodesis in patients with spinal tumors is a significant challenge. Although fusion is typically performed following spinal instrumentation to enhance stability, the environment in metastatic spine conditions is often suboptimal for fusion [1,3,5,7–9]. Factors such as poor bone quality, the impact of adjuvant therapies, and the typically short survival time of these patients complicate the fusion process [2,3]. Consequently, many clinicians opt for instrumentation alone without performing additional fusion after decompression, to provide immediate stability without the burden of achieving long-term bone fusion. Yee et al. reported that the fusion rate in patients with spinal metastatic tumors was only 28% [6], underscoring the difficulty of achieving successful arthrodesis in this population.

Although this approach can mitigate some immediate surgical challenges, it is associated with risks. The overall implant failure rate for these procedures ranges from approximately 3% to 13.8% [1,5]. Despite previous investigations of implant failure rates in patients with spinal metastatic tumors, the specific risk factors contributing to mechanical failure remain largely unknown. Considering the extended survival times of some patients owing to advances in cancer treatment, identifying these risk factors has become increasingly important [10–12].

This study aimed to determine the incidence of mechanical failure following decompression and fixation surgery in patients with metastatic spinal tumors. Additionally, we identified and analyzed the risk factors associated with such mechanical failures. Gaining this understanding is crucial for improving surgical outcomes and optimizing the management of spinal metastases in this challenging patient population.

2. Materials and Methods

2.1. Study Design and Patients

This study was approved by the institutional review board (IRB number: S2023-0763-0001, approved on 29 March 2023). The requirement for informed consent was waived owing to the retrospective nature of the study. This study was designed and reported in accordance with the Strengthening the Reporting of Observational Studies in Epidemiology (STROBE) statement for cohort studies. Between 2014 and 2020, 220 patients with spinal tumors who underwent decompression and instrumentation surgery, without fusion, for metastatic spinal tumors were enrolled in this study. Two experienced spine surgeons (JHC and JWP) performed all surgeries at a single institution. The primary indications for surgery included severe pain or neurological deterioration resulting from pathologic fractures or metastatic spinal cord compression [10,13].

The exclusion criteria were as follows: use of a fusion substrate during surgery; incomplete medical records, clinical scores, or radiographs; loss to follow-up or death within 6 months postoperatively; and surgery without instrumentation, including procedures such as cementing or decompression alone. After applying these exclusion criteria, the remaining patients were subjected to propensity score matching (PSM) based on preoperative variables such as age, sex, and bone mineral density (BMD) [14]. PSM was implemented to minimize selection bias and ensure comparability between the failure (F) and non-failure (non-F) groups. This matching resulted in a cohort with a 1:3 ratio that included 24 and 72 patients in the F and non-F groups, respectively. Thus, well-aligned groups were created for subsequent analyses.

2.2. Variables

A comprehensive set of variables was analyzed to assess the factors related to mechanical failure after instrumentation without fusion in patients with spinal tumors. These variables included demographic factors, tumor-related factors, and radiological assessments.

2.3. Demographic Factors

We collected data on age, sex, height, body mass index (BMI), and BMD from all patients enrolled. Additionally, we documented the type of surgery performed, including the number of laminectomy levels, fixation levels, screws placed in the tumor, the number of rods, and the use of cemented screws. We also tracked the time to mechanical failure, incidence of symptomatic local recurrence, and rate of reoperation to provide insights into the durability of surgical interventions.

2.4. Tumor-Related Factors

The origin of the tumor (e.g., lung, breast, or kidney) and the extent of tumor involvement, which included the number of vertebral levels affected by metastasis and whether the tumor had spread from the spinal column to other regions, were recorded. The number of vertebral levels instrumented above and below the affected area was also documented, typically involving two levels above and below the tumor-affected vertebrae.

2.5. Radiological Assessment

Radiological assessment was a critical component of this study. Hounsfield units (HUs) were measured on preoperative computed tomography (CT) scans to evaluate bone quality [15,16]. HU measurements were taken at specific vertebral levels, including the upper instrumented vertebra (UIV) and lowest instrumented vertebra (LIV). HU values were obtained by averaging the measurements across three axial slices of the vertebral body (VB), avoiding the cortical bone and focusing on the trabecular bone (Figure 1) [17]. Additional radiological factors such as Bilsky grades, spinal instability neoplastic scores (SINSs), and the extent of VB collapse were also assessed [12,18].

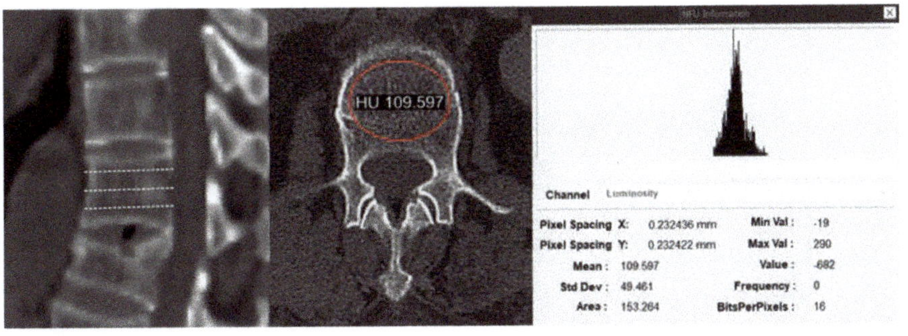

Figure 1. Preoperative computed tomography scan illustrating the method for measuring Hounsfield units (HUs) at the vertebral body. HU measurements were obtained from the trabecular bone at the upper and lowest instrumented vertebrae, represented by dashed lines indicating three axial slices per vertebra for accurate assessment.

2.6. Mechanical Failures

Mechanical failure of the instrumentation was defined based on clinical experience at our institution and established research criteria. Instrumentation failure was characterized by screw loosening, rod fracture or displacement, and subsidence of the cage, cement, or bone [19].

2.7. Statistical Analysis

Statistical analyses were conducted to identify the factors associated with mechanical failure. Logistic regression analysis was used to identify independent predictors of mechanical failure due to its suitability for binary outcome variables. Receiver operating characteristic (ROC) curve analysis was employed to determine the optimal cutoff for Hounsfield unit values, as this method provides sensitivity and specificity estimates. A Kaplan–Meier survival analysis was conducted to compare time-to-event outcomes between groups, providing insights into implant survival over time. In addition to propensity score matching, multivariate analyses included adjustments for confounding factors such as age, body mass index, and preoperative radiotherapy to further enhance the robustness of our findings. All statistical analyses were performed using IBM SPSS Statistics version 21.0 for Windows (IBM Corp., Armonk, NY, USA). Statistical significance was set at $p < 0.05$.

3. Results

3.1. Demographic Characteristics

The PSM resulted in a balanced distribution of covariates between the F and non-F groups, comprising 24 and 72 patients, respectively, achieving a 1:3 ratio. Specifically, the mean age difference between the groups was reduced from 4.22 years pre-matching to 0.61 years post-matching. No significant differences in age, sex, BMI, BMD, number of vertebral bodies involved, mode of surgery, PreopRT, major organ involvement, number of other bone lesions, or postoperative RT were observed between the two groups. The F group had a longer mean follow-up period than the non-F group (21.6 ± 18.8 vs. 15.4 ± 15.8 months), although this difference was not significant (p = 0.121, Table 1). The demographic and clinical characteristics of the 24 patients in the F group are shown in Table 2. The table outlines key factors, such as tumor origin, location, mode of surgery, number of laminectomies, fixation levels, screws placed in the tumor, and the type and timing of implant failures. The time to failure among the patients ranged from 0.25 to 27 months. Implant failure resulted from screw loosening (16 cases), rod breakage (2 cases), and cage subsidence. A significant proportion of patients (79.2%) in the F group required reoperation because of symptomatic implant failure.

Table 1. Demographic data of the mechanical failure and non-mechanical failure groups.

	Non-F Group	F Group	p
	(n = 72)	(n = 24)	
Age	58.4 ± 12.9	57.8 ± 13.1	0.856
Sex			1
Male	44 (61.1%)	14 (58.3%)	
Female	28 (38.9%)	10 (41.7%)	
Height	164.8 ± 9.5	166.6 ± 8.6	0.404
Weight	61.9 ± 10.3	64.7 ± 11.1	0.275
BMI	23.9 ± 6.5	23.3 ± 3.9	0.630
BMD	−1.9 ± 1.5	−2.1 ± 1.9	0.721
Follow-up period (months)	15.4 ± 15.8	21.6 ± 18.8	0.121
Involved vertebral bodies			0.731
1	27 (36.1%)	8 (33.3%)	
2	9 (12.5%)	5 (20.8%)	
≥3	36 (50.0%)	11 (45.8%)	
Pathologic fracture	53 (73.6%)	19 (79.2%)	0.785
Number of other bone lesions	1.1 ± 1.9	1.5 ± 3.5	0.551
Major organ metastasis	44 (61.1%)	17 (70.9%)	0.529
Mode of surgery			0.701
Fixation only	5 (6.9%)	1 (4.2%)	
Decompression and fixation	46 (63.9%)	14 (58.3%)	
Corpectomy and fixation	21 (29.2%)	9 (37.5%)	
PreopRT	24 (33.3%)	13 (54.2%)	0.115
PostopRT	50 (69.4%)	18 (75.0%)	0.795

BMI, body mass index; BMD, bone mineral density; RT, radiotherapy.

Table 2. Demographic and clinical summary of instrumentation failures in 24 patients.

Case No.	Sex/Age	Tumor Origin	Location	Mode of Surgery	No. of Laminectomy	Fixation Levels	Screws in Tumor	Failure Type	Time for Failure (Months)	Reoperation
1	M/50	Kidney	T5	Decompression and fixation	1	4	0	Failure c tumor recur	12	Yes
2	F/36	Breast	T12–L1	Fixation only	0	6	12	Failure	6	Yes
3	F/59	Lung	T12	Decompression and fixation	2	5	6	Failure c tumor recur	27	Yes
4	F/48	Kidney	T4	Corpectomy and fixation	1	4	0	Failure c tumor recur	17	Yes
5	M/57	Liver	C2	Decompression and fixation	1	2	0	Failure	1	Yes
6	M/71	Chondrosarcoma	T11	Corpectomy and fixation	2	4	1	Failure c tumor recur	1	Yes
7	M/72	Bladder	L3	Corpectomy and fixation	3	2.5	3	Failure c fracture	1	No
8	F/71	Kidney	T6	Corpectomy and fixation	1	4	0	Failure	2	Yes
9	M/71	MUO	L3–4	Decompression and fixation	3	4	0	Failure c tumor recur	10	Yes
10	F/27	Chondrosarcoma	T9	Decompression and fixation	5	2.5	0	Failure c fracture	0.25	Yes
11	F/47	Breast	L1	Decompression and fixation	1	2.5	3	Failure c tumor recur	2	No
12	F/56	Lung	L2,3	Decompression and fixation	3	3	1	Failure c fracture	2	Yes
13	M/75	Lung	L4	Decompression and fixation	2	2.5	1	Failure	3	No
14	F/60	Lung	L2–3	Decompression and fixation	2	5	5	Failure c tumor recur	14	Yes
15	F/72	Lung	T11–L1	Corpectomy and fixation	4	6	2	Failure	6	No
16	M/69	HCC	T11	Corpectomy and fixation	0	2	0	Failure c tumor recur	5	Yes
17	M/49	Lung	T8–9	Decompression and fixation	3	5	2	Failure c fracture	3	Yes
18	M/70	Liver	T10	Corpectomy and fixation	2	4	0	Failure c fracture	14	No
19	F/40	Breast	L4	Decompression and fixation	2	6	4	Failure	6	Yes
20	M/44	Thymus	T9	Corpectomy and fixation	3	5	0	Failure c fracture	18	Yes
21	M/63	Kidney	L4	Decompression and fixation	1	4	0	Rod breakage	14	Yes
22	M/70	Lung	L5	Decompression and fixation	1	4.5	3	Failure	5	Yes
23	M/56	Prostate	L3	Decompression and fixation	1	6	4	Failure	3	Yes
24	M/55	Lung	L1	Corpectomy and fixation	1	4	0	Rod breakage	26	Yes

M, male; F, female; MUO, metastasis of unknown origin; HCC, hepatocellular carcinoma; c, with.

3.2. Radiological Characteristics

Radiological characteristics, including the Bilsky grade, SINS, and VB collapse, were compared between the two groups (Table 3). No significant differences in the Bilsky grade, specific components of the SINS, or HU measurements at the UIV were identified between the two groups. However, the HU measurements at the LIV were significantly lower in the F group than in the non-F group (142.2 ± 62.2 vs. 178.9 ± 84.5, $p = 0.042$).

Table 3. Characteristics of the mechanical failure and non-mechanical failure groups.

	Non-F Group (n = 72)	F Group (n = 24)	p
Bilsky grade			0.312
0	2 (2.8%)	3 (12.5%)	
1	8 (11.1%)	3 (12.5%)	
2	20 (27.8%)	6 (25.0%)	
3	42 (58.3%)	12 (50.0%)	
SINS	10.3 ± 3.5	11.4 ± 3.0	0.208
Location			0.21
Semi-rigid	29 (40.3%)	7 (29.2%)	
Mobile spine	12 (16.7%)	8 (33.3%)	
Junctional	31 (43.1%)	9 (37.5%)	
Pain			0.699
Pain-free	7 (9.7%)	1 (4.3%)	
Occasional but not mechanical	16 (22.2%)	6 (26.1%)	
Yes	49 (68.1%)	16 (69.6%)	
Bone lesion			0.813
Blastic	10 (13.9%)	2 (8.3%)	
Mixed	7 (9.7%)	3 (12.5%)	
Lytic	55 (76.0%)	19 (79.2%)	
Alignment			0.627
Normal alignment	42 (58.3%)	13 (54.2%)	
De novo deformity	28 (38.9%)	11 (45.8%)	
Subluxation/translation	2 (2.8%)	0 (0.0%)	
VB collapse			0.652
None	11 (15.3%)	3 (12.5%)	
No collapse with >50% body involved	14 (19.4%)	4 (16.7%)	
<50% collapse	27 (37.5%)	7 (29.2%)	
>50% collapse	20 (27.8%)	10 (41.7%)	
Posterolateral involvement			0.82
None	8 (11.1%)	2 (8.3%)	
Unilateral	21 (29.2%)	9 (37.5%)	
Bilateral	43 (58.3%)	13 (54.2%)	
UIV HUs	191.1 ± 79.2	161.0 ± 58.5	0.115
LIV HUs	178.9 ± 84.5	142.2 ± 62.2	0.042 *

SINS, spinal instability neoplastic score; VB, vertebral body; UIV, upper instrumented vertebra; LIV, lower instrumented vertebra; HU, Hounsfield unit. * $p < 0.05$.

3.3. Surgical Characteristics

The surgical characteristics of the two groups are shown in Table 4. Although there were no significant differences in the levels of laminectomy, fixation, or the number of screws used between the two groups, the F group experienced a higher rate of symptomatic local recurrence (50.0% vs. 27.8%, $p = 0.08$) and a significantly higher rate of reoperation (79.2% vs. 33.3%, $p < 0.001$) than the non-F group.

Table 4. Surgical characteristics of the mechanical failure and non-mechanical failure groups.

	Non-F Group	F Group	p
	(n = 72)	(n = 24)	
Laminectomy levels	1.7 ± 1.2	1.9 ± 1.2	0.629
Fixation levels	3.7 ± 1.3	4.1 ± 1.3	0.279
Screws in tumor	1.0 ± 2.0	2.0 ± 2.8	0.139
No. of rods	2.0 ± 0.3	1.9 ± 0.2	0.503
No. of cemented screws	0.05 ± 0.4	0.2 ± 1.0	0.251
Symptomatic local recurrence	20 (27.8%)	12 (50.0%)	0.08
Time for symptomatic local recurrence	6.0 ± 8.4	9.6 ± 8.6	0.254
Reoperation	24 (33.3%)	19 (79.2%)	<0.001 *

No., number; * $p < 0.05$.

3.4. Logistic Regression and ROC Analyses

The logistic regression analysis revealed that lower LIV HU values and Bilsky grades were associated with an increased risk of mechanical failure (Table 5). Although other factors such as PreopRT and the SINS showed trends toward significance, they did not reach statistical significance in this study. However, the multivariate analysis identified lower LIV HU values as the only independent predictor of postoperative implant failure (p = 0.037). Furthermore, the ROC analysis (Figure 2) established a CT-measured LIV HU value < 127.27 as the cutoff value for predicting implant failure. This cutoff value had a sensitivity, specificity, and area under the curve of 69.6%, 73.6%, and 0.693, respectively (95% confidence interval: 0.55–0.83, p < 0.01). This finding was further confirmed by Kaplan–Meier survival analysis, indicating a significant difference in implant survival between the groups with LIV HU values above and below the cutoff (p = 0.0057, Figure 3).

Table 5. Logistic regression analysis for factors related with postoperative implant failure.

	Estimate	Std. Error	z Value	Pr (>|z|)	OR	lcl	ucl
Age	0.001	0.0178	0.06	0.956	1	0.97	1.04
BMI	−0.0178	0.0463	−0.39	0.7	0.98	0.88	1.06
PreopRT	0.8408	0.4753	1.77	0.077	2.32	0.92	5.99
Bilsky grade	−0.3424	0.2543	−1.35	0.178	0.71	0.43	1.18
SINS	0.0906	0.0759	1.19	0.233	1.09	0.95	1.28
Mode of surgery	0.3228	0.4231	0.76	0.445	1.38	0.6	3.21
Laminectomy levels	0.1114	0.1921	0.58	0.562	1.12	0.76	1.62
Fixation levels	0.1943	0.1765	1.1	0.271	1.21	0.86	1.73
No. of cemented screws	0.3574	0.3414	1.05	0.295	1.43	0.7	3.37
No. of rods	−0.5444	0.8247	−0.66	0.509	0.58	0.09	3.42
Screws in tumor	0.1778	0.0976	1.82	0.068	1.19	0.99	1.46
UIV HUs	−0.0059	0.0038	−1.54	0.124	0.99	0.99	1
LIV HUs	−0.0051	0.0036	−1.43	0.153	0.99	0.99	1
(Intercept)	1.3423	0.9957	1.35	0.178	3.83	0.58	30.49
Bilsky grade	−0.4757	0.2865	−1.66	0.097	0.62	0.35	1.09
LIV HUs	−0.01	0.0048	−2.08	0.037 *	0.99	0.98	1

Residual deviance/df = 80.3/78 = 1.03, pseudo-R^2 = 0.421 (Nagelkerke). BMI, body mass index; PreopRT, preoperative radiotherapy; SINS, spinal instability neoplastic score; No., number; UIV, upper instrumented vertebra; LIV, lower instrumented vertebra; HU, Hounsfield unit; OR, odds ratio; lcl, lower confidence limit; ucl, upper confidence limit. * p < 0.05.

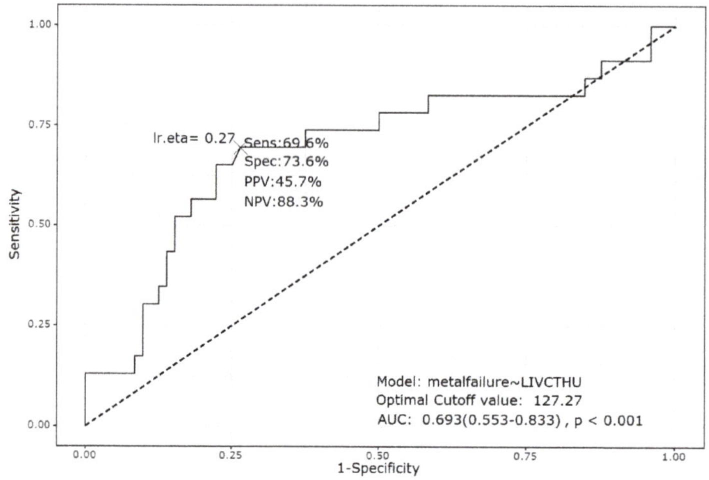

Figure 2. Receiver operating characteristic curve analysis for Hounsfield units (HUs) at the lowest instrumented vertebra (LIV), identifying a cutoff value of 127.273 for predicting mechanical failure after instrumentation without fusion. The analysis showed a sensitivity of 69.6% and a specificity of 73.6%, with an area under the curve (AUC) of 0.693 (95% confidence interval: 0.55–0.83) and $p < 0.001$. PPV, positive predictive value; NPV, negative predictive value.

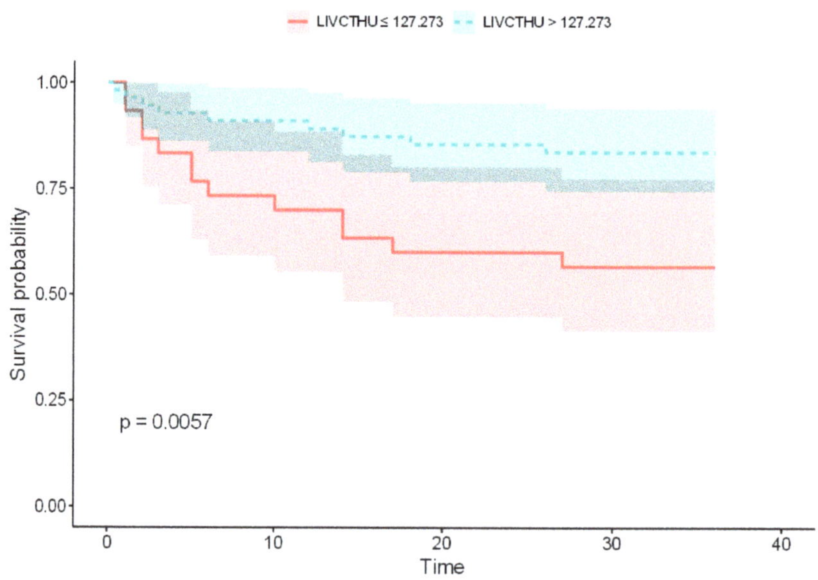

Figure 3. Kaplan–Meier survival curve comparing the time to mechanical failure between patients with Hounsfield unit (HU) values above and below the identified cutoff at the lowest instrumented vertebra (LIV). The survival curve demonstrates a significant difference in implant survival, with $p = 0.0057$, indicating that patients with LIV HU values < 127.273 have a higher risk of earlier mechanical failure.

3.5. Case Analysis

3.5.1. Case 1

A representative case from the F group was a 70-year-old male patient with liver cancer that had metastasized to the T10 vertebra (Figure 4). Preoperative CT imaging revealed an HU value of 94.15 at the LIV (T12) and 151.852 at the UIV. These values, particularly the LIV HUs, were below the identified cutoff value of 127.27, indicating an increased risk of implant failure. The patient underwent decompression with a partial corpectomy and percutaneous pedicle screw fixation from T8 to T12. Approximately 14 months postoperatively, the patient's back pain worsened, and CT tomography revealed a loosening of the T12 screws.

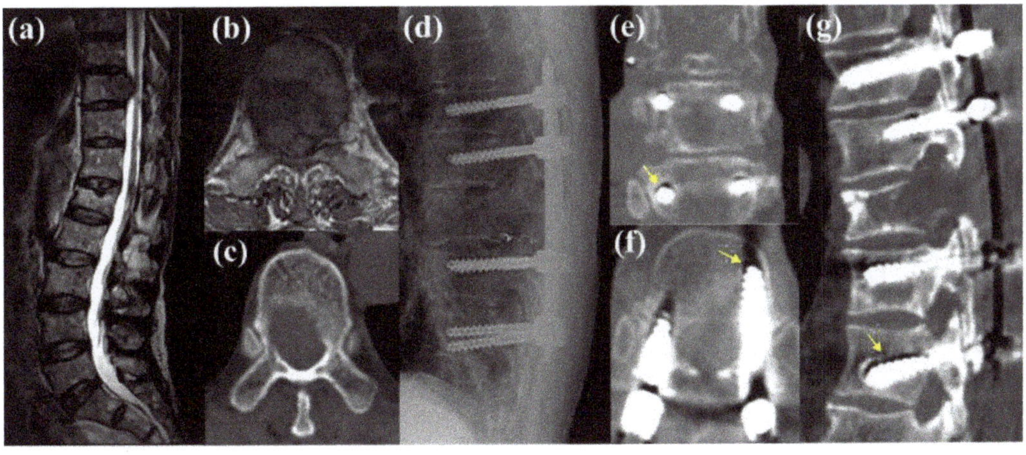

Figure 4. Representative case of a 70-year-old male patient with liver hepatocellular carcinoma metastasis to the T10 vertebra. (**a–c**) Preoperative magnetic resonance imaging and computed tomography (CT) imaging revealed the metastatic lesion, with a preoperative lowest instrumented vertebra Hounsfield unit value of 94.15, which is below the cutoff value associated with an increased risk of implant failure. (**d**) The patient underwent decompression with a partial corpectomy and posterior pedicle screw fixation from the T8 to T12. Postoperative plain radiographs initially showed an adequate hardware placement. (**e–g**) However, 14 months postoperatively, the patient experienced aggravated back pain, and subsequent CT imaging revealed loosening of the T12 pedicle screws (yellow arrows).

3.5.2. Case 2

Another failed case involved a 48-year-old female patient with renal cell carcinoma metastasis to the T4 vertebra (Figure 5). The patient underwent a T4 spondylectomy with mesh cage insertion and posterior fixation from T2 to T6. Preoperative CT imaging showed an average HU value of 264.862 at the UIV and 103.201 at the LIV, with the LIV HU below the cutoff value of 127.27. Approximately 17 months postoperatively, the patient experienced aggravated back pain, and CT tomography revealed loosening of the bilateral pedicle screws at the T6 vertebra. Consequently, revision surgery was performed, extending the fixation from C7 to T7.

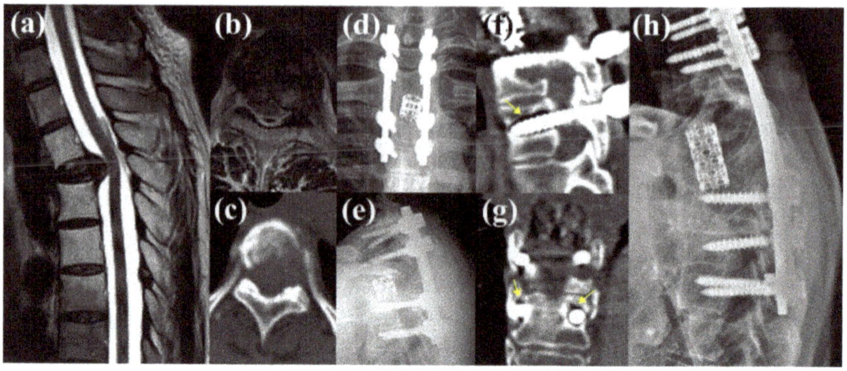

Figure 5. Case involving a 48-year-old female patient with renal cell carcinoma metastasis to the T4 vertebra. (**a–c**) Preoperative magnetic resonance imaging and computed tomography (CT) imaging revealed the metastatic lesion. (**d,e**) The patient underwent a T4 spondylectomy with mesh cage insertion and posterior fixation from T2 to T6. Preoperative computed tomography (CT) imaging showed an average Hounsfield unit value of 264.862 at the upper instrumented vertebra and 103.201 at the lowest instrumented vertebra. (**f,g**) Approximately 17 months postoperatively, the patient experienced aggravated back pain, and CT imaging revealed loosening of the bilateral pedicle screws at the T6 vertebra (yellow arrows), (**h**) leading to revision surgery extending the fixation from C7 to T7.

4. Discussion

This study aimed to identify risk factors associated with mechanical failure in patients undergoing instrumentation without fusion for metastatic spinal tumors. Among the various factors analyzed, lower HU values at the LIV were identified as a key predictor of implant failure. This result was consistent across multiple analyses, including logistic regression and Kaplan–Meier survival analyses, underscoring the critical role of bone quality, as measured by HUs, in the success of instrumentation without fusion in patients with metastatic spinal tumors.

The decision to perform instrumentation without fusion in these patients was influenced by several factors [1,6,10,11,20,21]. First, the average life expectancy of patients with spinal metastases is often limited to a few months, indicating that even with attempting fusion, patients frequently succumb to their illness before achieving bone union [4,7,22]. Second, the bone quality in these patients, particularly in the fusion bed, is often poor, thus further reducing the likelihood of successful fusion [5,6,12,23]. Previous studies have reported mixed outcomes for fixation alone [24]. Some studies have suggested that even in cases of rod fracture, patients may not always experience significant discomfort, implying that fixation alone might suffice [24]. However, other studies have indicated that additional stabilization efforts may be necessary to avoid complications. As patients' survival rates improve, concerns regarding the impact of spinal construct instability on the quality of life have also increased. In our study, 19 of the 24 patients in the F group (approximately 80%) required reoperation, highlighting the significant clinical burden of mechanical failure. Additionally, the time to symptomatic recurrence differed between the groups, with issues arising at an average of 6 months in the non-F group and 9.6 months in the F group. Complications related to spinal construct stability occurred within the expected survival period of these patients, making this an essential consideration for surgical planning.

The logistic regression analysis revealed that several factors were associated with implant failure after fixation-only surgery. PreopRT showed a trend toward significance (p = 0.077), with the placement of screws in areas of tumor involvement correlating with higher failure rates. However, factors such as the number of fixation levels and extent of laminectomy were not significantly associated with failure. Importantly, the multivariate analysis identified lower HU values at the LIV as the only independent predictor of failure. The ROC analysis determined a cutoff value of 127.27, below which the risk of implant-related failure due to weakened bone at the LIV was significantly increased. This finding was further confirmed by Kaplan–Meier survival analysis, where a significant difference ($p = 0.0057$) in survival rates between the groups with HU values above and below the cutoff was observed.

CT HU measurements are well established as predictive tools for implant failure in various spine surgeries [15,16], particularly in long-level deformity correction procedures [25–27]. In such surgeries, low HU values have been correlated with an increased risk of hardware-related complications, emphasizing the importance of bone quality assessment in surgical planning. Our study extends this knowledge to patients with metastatic spinal tumors, demonstrating that HU measurements at the LIV are critical in predicting the likelihood of implant failure. The identified cutoff value of 127.27 HUs provides a practical and clinically relevant threshold for assessing risk, further supporting the utility of CT HUs as a non-invasive predictor of surgical outcomes. Moreover, the predictive value of HU measurements for implant stability could have implications beyond spine surgery. For instance, in major joint replacement surgeries or other orthopedic procedures where bone quality significantly affects implant longevity, HU assessments could similarly aid in preoperative planning and risk stratification, potentially guiding the choice of stabilization techniques or implant materials [28,29].

One of the more intriguing findings of this study is the greater predictive power of LIV HU values than that of the UIV. Although both levels are crucial for maintaining spinal stability, the LIV may be more susceptible to mechanical failure than the UIV because of its position as the lower anchor point in the construct, where stress and load are maximized [5,30]. This finding aligns with those of studies in other contexts such as deformity correction, where the LIV plays a pivotal role in the overall integrity of the spinal construct [1,3,30]. For instance, in a study on degenerative lumbar scoliosis, Yuan et al. reported a loosening rate of 45.4% at the LIV compared to 17.7% at the UIV, suggesting that the primary cause of loosening was a weakened BMD at the LIV [31]. This observation is consistent with our findings, in which both representative cases (Figures 4 and 5) demonstrated lower HU values at the LIV than at the UIV, leading to screw loosening at the LIV. Although anatomical factors such as screw trajectory and insertion angle may also contribute to loosening, within the heterogeneity of metastatic spinal tumors, the HU value at the LIV was the most objective predictor of loosening. Previous studies on degenerative conditions have similarly highlighted the significance of HUs in screw trajectory and its impact on outcomes [15,16]. Therefore, ensuring adequate bone quality at the LIV is essential for the long-term success of spinal instrumentation, particularly in patients with compromised bone quality.

Considering the critical role of LIV HU values identified in this study, alternative strategies for patients with HU values below the identified threshold of 127.27 need to be determined. This study provides a reference to guide clinicians and surgeons in their decision-making processes. For patients expected to have long-term survival, and thus a prolonged need for stable spinal instrumentation [32], surgical techniques such as the use of cement-augmented screws, thicker screws, or longer screws extending into the anterior VB may be considered [10,33,34]. Cement-augmented pedicle screws, which improve pull-out strength and reduce the risk of fixation failure in patients with osteoporosis or spinal metastases, could be particularly beneficial [34,35]. Unfortunately, in our study, only an average of 0.2% of cemented screws per patient were used in the F group, highlighting a potential area for improvement in surgical techniques. Additionally, the use of fenestrated pedicle screws with cementation further reduces the risk of screw loosening, which was a significant concern in our study [35]. While cement augmentation provides improved purchase power and stability, it is not without risks [35,36]. Cement leakage into the foramen can lead to root symptoms by compressing nearby nerves, and the inadvertent entry of cement into the venous system poses a risk of venous thrombus formation, which could result in serious complications [21,35,37]. Therefore, a careful technique and thorough intraoperative monitoring are essential when using cement-augmented screws to mitigate these risks.

These strategies can mitigate the risk of mechanical failure in high-risk populations. Future research should focus on evaluating the effectiveness of these techniques in improving outcomes for patients with low HU values at the LIV, as well as exploring the integration of other advanced imaging modalities or bone augmentation techniques [16,33–35]. Currently, advanced imaging techniques being developed and applied in other orthopedic fields include quantitative computed tomography (Q-CT) with phantom calibration, which allows for standardized, quantitative bone density assessments, and an AI-based volumetric analysis that evaluates bone structure in three dimensions [38,39]. These methods may provide a more detailed and precise assessment of bone quality, beyond traditional HU measurements, and could significantly enhance predictive accuracy for implant stability in patients with a compromised bone integrity.

The strength of this study lies in its large cohort size of 220 patients, including a focused analysis of 24 patients in the F group, representing approximately 10% of the cohort. The use of PSM to create a 1:3 ratio between the F and non-F groups minimized bias and strengthened the validity of the findings. This methodological rigor suggests that the results are reliable and applicable to similar patient populations. However, this study has some limitations. First, the retrospective design inherently carries the risk of selection bias, and the relatively small sample size of the F group may have limited the generalizability of the findings. Given the initial disparity in sample sizes between the F group and non-F group, we implemented propensity score matching (PSM) to create balanced groups for meaningful comparisons. Despite this approach, the limited size of the failure group remains a constraint. Although the analysis within the F group was limited by its size, gathering this number of failure cases at a single institution is a significant achievement. Second, the cohort included patients with metastatic spinal tumors across different spinal regions (cervical, thoracic, and lumbar), introducing a degree of heterogeneity that could influence the outcomes. The biomechanical and anatomical differences between these regions may have affected the risk of mechanical failure, which was not fully accounted for in this study. Additionally, while this study focused on key factors such as HU values and mechanical failure, other potential contributors, such as the number of tumor-affected segments, the duration of internal fixation, and the use of postoperative external fixation, may also influence fixation stability. Furthermore, our post hoc power analysis indicated a statistical power of approximately 72% with the current sample size, which is below the commonly recommended threshold of 80%. Future studies with larger, multicenter cohorts could provide additional insights by analyzing different spinal regions separately, to confirm whether these findings hold consistently across the cervical, thoracic, and lumbar segments. Finally, although HU values provide a valuable assessment of bone quality, they do not encompass all aspects of bone health, such as microarchitectural integrity, which may also influence implant stability.

5. Conclusions

This study suggests that preoperative bone quality assessment using CT HU measurements at the LIV may help in predicting the risk of mechanical failure following spinal instrumentation without fusion in patients with metastatic spinal tumors. While the identified HU cutoff value of 127.27 could serve as a useful tool for risk stratification, it should be considered as part of a comprehensive assessment of patient-specific risk factors rather than a standalone predictor. Personalized surgical approaches, particularly for patients with compromised bone quality, may benefit from incorporating HU measurements into preoperative planning. Future research is encouraged to validate these findings in larger prospective cohorts and to explore alternative surgical strategies for high-risk patients.

Author Contributions: Conceptualization, J.H.C.; methodology, J.H.C. and S.Y.S.; software, D.W.C.; validation, J.H.C., S.K. and D.W.C.; formal analysis, S.Y.S.; investigation, H.R.L.; resources, J.H.Y.; data curation, H.R.L.; writing—original draft preparation, H.R.L.; writing—review and editing, J.H.C.; visualization, S.K.; supervision, J.H.C.; project administration, J.H.C.; funding acquisition, J.H.Y. All authors have read and agreed to the published version of the manuscript.

Funding: This research received no external funding.

Institutional Review Board Statement: This study was conducted in accordance with the Declaration of Helsinki and approved by the institutional review board of Seoul Asan Medical Center (protocol code S2023-0763-0001, approved on 29 March 2023).

Informed Consent Statement: Informed consent was waived due to the retrospective nature of the study.

Data Availability Statement: Data are available upon reasonable request.

Acknowledgments: We would like to thank the English editing service for improving the clarity and language of this manuscript.

Conflicts of Interest: The authors report no conflicts of interest concerning the materials or methods used in this study or the findings specified in this paper. No financial support was received for this study.

References

1. Hayashi, K.; Tsuchiya, H. The role of surgery in the treatment of metastatic bone tumor. *Int. J. Clin. Oncol.* **2022**, *27*, 1238–1246. [CrossRef]
2. Vrionis, F.D.; Small, J. Surgical management of metastatic spinal neoplasms. *Neurosurg. Focus* **2003**, *15*, E12. [CrossRef] [PubMed]
3. Healey, J.H.; Brown, H.K. Complications of bone metastases: Surgical management. *Cancer* **2000**, *88*, 2940–2951. [CrossRef]
4. Wu, X.; Ye, Z.; Pu, F.; Chen, S.; Wang, B.; Zhang, Z.; Yang, C.; Yang, S.; Shao, Z. Palliative Surgery in Treating Painful Metastases of the Upper Cervical Spine: Case Report and Review of the Literature. *Medicine* **2016**, *95*, e3558. [CrossRef] [PubMed]
5. Cai, Z.; Zhao, Y.; Tang, X.; Yang, R.; Yan, T.; Guo, W. Factors associated with spinal fixation mechanical failure after tumor resection: A systematic review and meta-analysis. *J. Orthop. Surg. Res.* **2022**, *17*, 110. [CrossRef]
6. Yee, T.J.; Saadeh, Y.S.; Strong, M.J.; Ward, A.L.; Elswick, C.M.; Srinivasan, S.; Park, P.; Oppenlander, M.E.; Spratt, D.E.; Jackson, W.C.; et al. Survival, fusion, and hardware failure after surgery for spinal metastatic disease. *J. Neurosurg. Spine* **2021**, *34*, 665–672. [CrossRef]
7. Liu, J.K.; Apfelbaum, R.I.; Schmidt, M.H. Surgical management of cervical spinal metastasis: Anterior reconstruction and stabilization techniques. *Neurosurg. Clin. N. Am.* **2004**, *15*, 413–424. [CrossRef] [PubMed]
8. Kim, G.U.; Park, W.T.; Chang, M.C.; Lee, G.W. Diagnostic Technology for Spine Pathology. *Asian Spine J.* **2022**, *16*, 764–775. [CrossRef]
9. Kim, Y.H.; Ha, K.Y.; Kim, Y.S.; Kim, K.W.; Rhyu, K.W.; Park, J.B.; Shin, J.H.; Kim, Y.Y.; Lee, J.S.; Park, H.Y.; et al. Lumbar Interbody Fusion and Osteobiologics for Lumbar Fusion. *Asian Spine J.* **2022**, *16*, 1022–1033. [CrossRef]
10. Park, S.J.; Park, J.S.; Lee, C.S.; Kang, B.J.; Jung, C.W. Trends in Survival and Surgical Methods in Patients Surgically Treated for Metastatic Spinal Tumors: 25-Year Experience in a Single Institution. *Clin. Orthop. Surg.* **2023**, *15*, 109–117. [CrossRef]
11. Shin, H.K.; Kim, M.; Lee, S.; Lee, J.J.; Park, D.; Jeon, S.R.; Roh, S.W.; Park, J.H. Surgical strategy for metastatic spinal tumor patients with surgically challenging situation. *Medicine* **2022**, *101*, e29560. [CrossRef]
12. Rothrock, R.J.; Barzilai, O.; Reiner, A.S.; Lis, E.; Schmitt, A.M.; Higginson, D.S.; Yamada, Y.; Bilsky, M.H.; Laufer, I. Survival Trends After Surgery for Spinal Metastatic Tumors: 20-Year Cancer Center Experience. *Neurosurgery* **2021**, *88*, 402–412. [CrossRef] [PubMed]
13. Galgano, M.; Fridley, J.; Oyelese, A.; Telfian, A.; Kosztowski, T.; Choi, D.; Gokaslan, Z.L. Surgical management of spinal metastases. *Expert Rev. Anticancer. Ther.* **2018**, *18*, 463–472. [CrossRef] [PubMed]
14. Kane, L.T.; Fang, T.; Galetta, M.S.; Goyal, D.K.C.; Nicholson, K.J.; Kepler, C.K.; Vaccaro, A.R.; Schroeder, G.D. Propensity Score Matching: A Statistical Method. *Clin. Spine Surg.* **2020**, *33*, 120–122. [CrossRef] [PubMed]
15. Zou, D.; Muheremu, A.; Sun, Z.; Zhong, W.; Jiang, S.; Li, W. Computed tomography Hounsfield unit-based prediction of pedicle screw loosening after surgery for degenerative lumbar spine disease. *J. Neurosurg. Spine* **2020**, *32*, 716–721. [CrossRef]
16. Sakai, Y.; Takenaka, S.; Matsuo, Y.; Fujiwara, H.; Honda, H.; Makino, T.; Kaito, T. Hounsfield unit of screw trajectory as a predictor of pedicle screw loosening after single level lumbar interbody fusion. *J. Orthop. Sci.* **2018**, *23*, 734–738. [CrossRef] [PubMed]
17. Courtois, E.C.; Ohnmeiss, D.D.; Guyer, R.D. Assessing lumbar vertebral bone quality: A methodological evaluation of CT and MRI as alternatives to traditional DEXA. *Eur. Spine J.* **2023**, *32*, 3176–3182. [CrossRef]
18. Fisher, C.G.; Schouten, R.; Versteeg, A.L.; Boriani, S.; Varga, P.P.; Rhines, L.D.; Kawahara, N.; Fourney, D.; Weir, L.; Reynolds, J.J. Reliability of the Spinal Instability Neoplastic Score (SINS) among radiation oncologists: An assessment of instability secondary to spinal metastases. *Radiat. Oncol.* **2014**, *9*, 69. [CrossRef]

19. Jacobs, E.; van Royen, B.J.; van Kuijk, S.M.; Merk, J.M.; Stadhouder, A.; van Rhijn, L.W.; Willems, P.C. Prediction of mechanical complications in adult spinal deformity surgery—The GAP score versus the Schwab classification. *Spine J.* **2019**, *19*, 781–788. [CrossRef]
20. Carrwik, C.; Olerud, C.; Robinson, Y. Survival after surgery for spinal metastatic disease: A nationwide multiregistry cohort study. *BMJ Open* **2021**, *11*, e049198. [CrossRef]
21. Hong, S.H.; Chang, B.S.; Kim, H.; Kang, D.H.; Chang, S.Y. An Updated Review on the Treatment Strategy for Spinal Metastasis from the Spine Surgeon's Perspective. *Asian Spine J.* **2022**, *16*, 799–811. [CrossRef] [PubMed]
22. Amankulor, N.M.; Xu, R.; Iorgulescu, J.B.; Chapman, T.; Reiner, A.S.; Riedel, E.; Lis, E.; Yamada, Y.; Bilsky, M.; Laufer, I. The incidence and patterns of hardware failure after separation surgery in patients with spinal metastatic tumors. *Spine J.* **2014**, *14*, 1850–1859. [CrossRef]
23. Groenen, K.H.; Pouw, M.H.; Hannink, G.; Hosman, A.J.; van der Linden, Y.M.; Verdonschot, N.; Tanck, E. The effect of radiotherapy, and radiotherapy combined with bisphosphonates or RANK ligand inhibitors on bone quality in bone metastases. A systematic review. *Radiother. Oncol.* **2016**, *119*, 194–201. [CrossRef] [PubMed]
24. Park, S.J.; Lee, K.H.; Lee, C.S.; Jung, J.Y.; Park, J.H.; Kim, G.L.; Kim, K.T. Instrumented surgical treatment for metastatic spinal tumors: Is fusion necessary? *J. Neurosurg. Spine* **2020**, *32*, 456–464. [CrossRef]
25. Yao, Y.C.; Chao, H.; Kao, K.Y.; Lin, H.H.; Wang, S.T.; Chang, M.C.; Liu, C.L.; Chou, P.H. CT Hounsfield unit is a reliable parameter for screws loosening or cages subsidence in minimally invasive transforaminal lumbar interbody fusion. *Sci. Rep.* **2023**, *13*, 1620. [CrossRef]
26. Shu, L.; Wang, X.; Li, L.; Aili, A.; Zhang, R.; Liu, W.; Muheremu, A. Computed Tomography-Based Prediction of Lumbar Pedicle Screw Loosening. *Biomed. Res. Int.* **2023**, *2023*, 8084597. [CrossRef] [PubMed]
27. Li, D.; Sun, C.; Jiang, J.; Lu, F.; Xia, X.; Wang, H.; Zou, F.; Ma, X. A study of screw placement to obtain the optimal pull-out resistance of lumbar pedicle screws-analysis of Hounsfield units measurements based on computed tomography. *BMC Musculoskelet. Disord.* **2022**, *23*, 124. [CrossRef]
28. Nishi, M.; Okano, I.; Yoshikawa, Y.; Tochio, H.; Usui, Y.; Inagaki, K. Relationship Between Acetabular Hounsfield Unit Values and Periprosthetic Fractures in Cementless Total Hip Arthroplasty: A Matched Case-Control Study. *Arthroplast. Today* **2022**, *14*, 216–222.e211. [CrossRef]
29. Ishibashi, S.; Nakasa, T.; Ikuta, Y.; Kawabata, S.; Moriwaki, D.; Sakurai, S.; Adachi, N. The Hounsfield Unit Values of Talar Subchondral Bone Predict Articular Cartilage Degeneration in Patients with Ankle Osteoarthritis. *Foot Ankle Int.* **2024**, *45*, 1292–1301. [CrossRef]
30. Tse, C.B.; Mandler, S.I.; Crawford, H.A.; Field, A.J.F. Risk factors for distal construct failure in posterior spinal instrumented fusion for adolescent idiopathic scoliosis: A retrospective cohort study. *Spine Deform.* **2023**, *11*, 1169–1176. [CrossRef]
31. Yuan, L.; Zhang, X.; Zeng, Y.; Chen, Z.; Li, W. Incidence, Risk, and Outcome of Pedicle Screw Loosening in Degenerative Lumbar Scoliosis Patients Undergoing Long-Segment Fusion. *Glob. Spine J.* **2023**, *13*, 1064–1071. [CrossRef] [PubMed]
32. Tan, K.A.; Tan, J.H.; Zaw, A.S.; Tan, J.Y.H.; Hey, H.W.D.; Kumar, N. Evaluation of Prognostic Factors and Proposed Changes to the Modified Tokuhashi Score in Patients with Spinal Metastases from Breast Cancer. *Spine* **2018**, *43*, 512–519. [CrossRef] [PubMed]
33. Viezens, L.; Sellenschloh, K.; Püschel, K.; Morlock, M.M.; Lehmann, W.; Huber, G.; Weiser, L. Impact of Screw Diameter on Pedicle Screw Fatigue Strength-A Biomechanical Evaluation. *World Neurosurg.* **2021**, *152*, e369–e376. [CrossRef] [PubMed]
34. Moussazadeh, N.; Rubin, D.G.; McLaughlin, L.; Lis, E.; Bilsky, M.H.; Laufer, I. Short-segment percutaneous pedicle screw fixation with cement augmentation for tumor-induced spinal instability. *Spine J.* **2015**, *15*, 1609–1617. [CrossRef]
35. Barzilai, O.; McLaughlin, L.; Lis, E.; Reiner, A.S.; Bilsky, M.H.; Laufer, I. Utility of Cement Augmentation via Percutaneous Fenestrated Pedicle Screws for Stabilization of Cancer-Related Spinal Instability. *Oper. Neurosurg.* **2019**, *16*, 593–599. [CrossRef]
36. Elder, B.D.; Lo, S.F.; Holmes, C.; Goodwin, C.R.; Kosztowski, T.A.; Lina, I.A.; Locke, J.E.; Witham, T.F. The biomechanics of pedicle screw augmentation with cement. *Spine J.* **2015**, *15*, 1432–1445. [CrossRef]
37. Morimoto, T.; Kobayashi, T.; Hirata, H.; Tsukamoto, M.; Yoshihara, T.; Toda, Y.; Mawatari, M. Cardiopulmonary Cement Embolism Following Cement-Augmented Pedicle Screw Fixation: A Narrative Review. *Medicina* **2023**, *59*, 407. [CrossRef]
38. Kulkarni, A.G.; Thonangi, Y.; Pathan, S.; Gunjotikar, S.; Goparaju, P.; Talwar, I.; Jaggi, S.; Shah, S.; Shah, N.; Kursija, G. Should Q-CT Be the Gold Standard for Detecting Spinal Osteoporosis? *Spine* **2022**, *47*, E258–E264. [CrossRef]
39. Lee, Y.S.; Hong, N.; Witanto, J.N.; Choi, Y.R.; Park, J.; Decazes, P.; Eude, F.; Kim, C.O.; Chang Kim, H.; Goo, J.M.; et al. Deep neural network for automatic volumetric segmentation of whole-body CT images for body composition assessment. *Clin. Nutr.* **2021**, *40*, 5038–5046. [CrossRef]

Journal of
Clinical Medicine

MDPI

Systematic Review

Artificial Intelligence Models for Predicting Outcomes in Spinal Metastasis: A Systematic Review and Meta-Analysis

Vivek Sanker [1,*], Prachi Dawer [2], Alexander Thaller [3], Zhikai Li [4], Philip Heesen [5], Srinath Hariharan [1], Emil O. R. Nordin [1], Maria Jose Cavagnaro [1], John Ratliff [1] and Atman Desai [1]

1 Department of Neurosurgery, Stanford University, Palo Alto, CA 94305, USA; hsrinath@stanford.edu (S.H.); enordin@stanford.edu (E.O.R.N.); mjcava@stanford.edu (M.J.C.); jratliff@stanford.edu (J.R.); atman@stanford.edu (A.D.)
2 Department of Neurosurgery, University College of Medical Sciences, New Delhi 110095, India; prachidawar59@gmail.com
3 Department of Neurosurgery, Medical University of Graz, 8010 Graz, ST, Austria; alexander.thaller@medunigraz.at
4 Department of Clinical Neurosciences, Addenbrooke's Hospital, Cambridge CB2 0QQ, UK; zl498@cam.ac.uk
5 Faculty of Medicine, University of Zurich, 8006 Zurich, Switzerland; heesenphilip99@gmail.com
* Correspondence: vsanker@stanford.edu

Abstract: Background: Spinal metastases can cause significant impairment of neurological function and quality of life. Hence, personalized clinical decision-making based on prognosis and likely outcome is desirable. The effectiveness of AI in predicting complications and treatment outcomes for patients with spinal metastases is assessed. **Methods:** A thorough search was carried out through the PubMed, Scopus, Web of Science, Embase, and Cochrane databases up until 27 January 2025. Included were studies that used AI-based models to predict outcomes for adult patients with spinal metastases. Three reviewers independently extracted the data, and screening was conducted in accordance with PRISMA principles. AUC results were pooled using a random-effects model, and the PROBAST program was used to evaluate the study's quality. **Results:** Included were 47 articles totaling 25,790 patients. For training, internal validation, and external validation, the weighted average AUCs were 0.762, 0.876, and 0.810, respectively. The Skeletal Oncology Research Group machine learning algorithms (SORG-MLAs) were the ones externally validated the most, continuously producing AUCs > 0.84 for 90-day and 1-year mortality. Models based on radiomics showed promise in preoperative planning, especially for outcomes of radiation and concealed blood loss. Most research concentrated on breast, lung, and prostate malignancies, which limited its applicability to less common tumors. **Conclusions:** AI models have shown reasonable accuracy in predicting mortality, ambulatory status, blood loss, and surgical complications in patients with spinal metastases. Wider implementation necessitates additional validation, data standardization, and ethical and regulatory framework evaluation. Future work should concentrate on creating multimodal, hybrid models and assessing their practical applications.

Keywords: artificial intelligence; machine learning; deep learning; spine metastasis; complications

1. Introduction

The spine is one of the most common sites of metastasis, after the lung and the liver. In patients with systemic cancer, approximately more than half develop spinal metastases, and approximately 10% are symptomatic [1]. Surgery can significantly improve quality of life in selected patients [2], and overall treatments have advanced in recent years to enhance overall clinical results and survival [3]. However, the likelihood of good outcomes must always be weighed against the risks of complications and the economic costs in each individual case [4].

Artificial intelligence (AI) is emerging as a potentially powerful tool to enhance clinical decision-making through analysis of large datasets to predict individual patient outcomes and risks, through machine learning and deep learning algorithms.

This systematic review's main goal was to assess the state of artificial intelligence (AI) models created to forecast outcomes and problems for patients who have spinal metastases. The degree to which these models included explainability and interpretability—two crucial components for clinical confidence and the practical application of AI tools—was specifically examined in addition to summarizing performance measures. The following definition of the primary clinical outcomes was made to guarantee uniformity between studies:

- Survival: At the longest or most precise follow-up available, it is reported as either overall survival (OS) or progression-free survival (PFS). PFS is the period of time until disease progression or death, whereas OS is the period of time from diagnosis or the start of therapy to death from any cause.
- Ambulatory status: Usually classified as either ambulatory or non-ambulatory, this refers to the patient's capacity to walk on their own or with the use of assistive technology.
- Complications: Contains any unfavorable events that occur during or after surgery, such as bleeding, infection, thrombosis, or neurological decline. Standard classification systems (e.g., Clavien–Dindo) were used to stratify these by severity whenever possible.

2. Materials and Methods

2.1. Ethical Review

Ethical review and approval were waived for this study due to it being a systematic review of previously published data that did not involve human participants or the collection of new data.

2.2. Search Strategy

We searched PubMed, Scopus, Web of Science Advance, Cochrane, and Embase (Ovid) databases to identify relevant studies, using a search query with specific keywords like 'spine metastases', 'artificial intelligence', 'machine learning', 'deep learning', and 'outcomes' (Supplementary Table S1). The population under consideration included adults with spinal metastases. The objective was to identify studies reporting the use of AI/deep learning (DL) models in predicting treatment and outcome prediction in spinal metastases [5].

Irrelevant articles, such as studies unrelated to spinal metastases and those purely investigating primary spinal tumors, were excluded. Animal studies, reviews, and non-original research articles were also excluded from our analysis to ensure the inclusion of primary research data relevant to our objective. The electronic search ranged from the period's earliest available date up to 27 January 2025 [5].

2.3. Screening of Studies

Each study's title and abstract were screened for relevance before proceeding to full-text screening, which was independently assessed by two reviewers (PD and VS). Any discrepancies were addressed through consultation with a third reviewer (SH). This review adhered to the PRISMA (Preferred Reporting Items for Systematic Reviews and Meta-

Analyses) guidelines but was not registered on the PROSPERO international prospective register of systematic reviews (Figure 1).

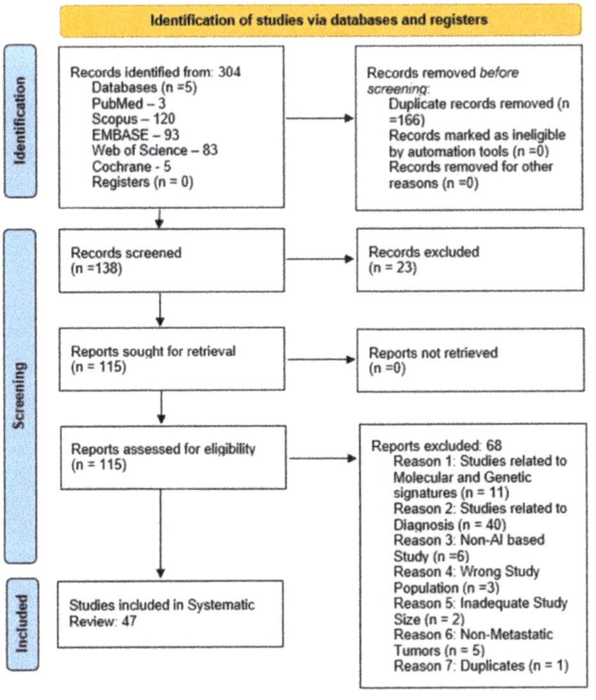

Figure 1. A PRISMA flow diagram is presented to illustrate the screening of studies.

2.4. Data Extraction

Three independent authors (PD, VS, and AT) extracted relevant data from the included studies. The data collected included study design, participant demographics, and the number of participants with respective outcomes and complications. Discrepancies in data extraction were resolved through consensus [5].

2.5. Data Analysis

Relevant variables were extracted from each of the included articles, such as the primary tumor type, cohort size, and prediction model performance matrices: area under the receiver operating characteristic curve (AUC) and type of validation (internal or external validation). The weighted average of the AUC was calculated. All statistical analyses were conducted using Excel, R Statistical Software, version 4.3.1, and Python, version 3.13.3.

We conducted a random-effects meta-analysis using restricted maximum likelihood (REML) estimation to account for both within-study and between-study variability. This approach assumes that the true effect size may vary across studies due to underlying differences in study populations, methodologies, or settings. REML was used to estimate the between-study variance (τ^2), providing an unbiased and efficient estimate of heterogeneity. Pooled effect estimates were calculated as weighted averages of the individual study effects, with weights derived from both the within-study variance and the estimated between-study variance. The Standardized Mean Difference (SMD) along with the 95% confidence interval (CI) was used to compare continuous performance metrics like AUC between studies after having a pooled estimate.

2.6. Quality Assessment

The quality assessment was performed using the PROBAST (Prediction model Risk of Bias Assessment Tool (Supplementary Figures S1 and S2).

PROBAST is designed for assessing the risk of bias and applicability in studies that develop, validate, or update predictive models. It is a structured tool that assesses four domains:

Participants: evaluating whether the data sources or patient samples used for training and testing are appropriate and representative of the clinical population. Predictors: ensuring that input data or predictors are well defined and appropriately measured. Outcome: ensuring that the outcomes (e.g., model predictions, decisions) are clearly defined and relevant to clinical scenarios. Analysis: evaluating whether the model performance metrics, training/validation processes, and statistical analysis methods are robust and unbiased.

In the Participants Section, 32 studies were flagged as having low risk of bias (68%), whilst 15 studies were flagged as having unclear risk/some concerns (32%). In the Predictors Section, 23 studies were flagged as having low risk of bias (49%), 16 studies flagged as having unclear risk/some concerns (34%), and 8 studies flagged as having high risk (17%). In the Outcome Section, 18 studies were flagged as having low risk of bias (38%), 16 as having unclear risk/some concerns (34%), and 13 as having high risk (28%). In the Analysis Section, 3 studies were flagged as having low risk of bias (6%), 15 studies flagged as having unclear risk/some concerns (32%), and 29 flagged as having high risk (62%).

3. Results

This review encompasses 47 studies published between 2016 and 2025, including a total of 26,038 patients with a median of 269 patients per study, ranging from 30 to 2786 patients (Table 1).

Table 1. An overview of the studies analyzed is presented.

Year of publishing (range)	2016–2025
Total number of patients	25,790
Median number of patients	268
Number of patients per study (range)	30–2786

Among the 47 studies, the three most common primary tumor types were breast cancer, lung cancer and prostate cancer, reported in 33 (70.2%), 32 (68.1%), and 23 (48.9%) studies, respectively (Table 2 and Figure 2). In contrast, neuroendocrine tumors, bladder cancer and esophageal cancer were the least common, each reported in three (6.4%), three (6.4%), and four (8.5%) studies, respectively (Table 2).

Five of the forty-seven studies reported AUC values for the established models during training of the model (Table 3), eighteen for internal validation (Table 4), and fourteen for external validation (Table 5).

The weighted average AUC value among the five studies that reported AUC values and corresponding 95% confidence intervals for the training of the established models is 0.762 (95% CI: 0.704–0.717). Wherever 95% confidence intervals were not reported, the weighted average of the reported 95% confidence intervals was used.

Table 2. The frequency of primary tumor types is shown. Studies analyzing multiple primary tumor types have been included in all applicable categories.

Primary Tumor Type	Number of Studies (Percentage)
Breast cancer	33/47 (70.2%)
Lung cancer	32/47 (68.1%)
Prostate cancer	23/47 (48.9%)
Esophageal cancer	4/47 (8.5%)
Bladder cancer	3/47 (6.4%)
Neuroendocrine tumors	3/47 (6.4%)

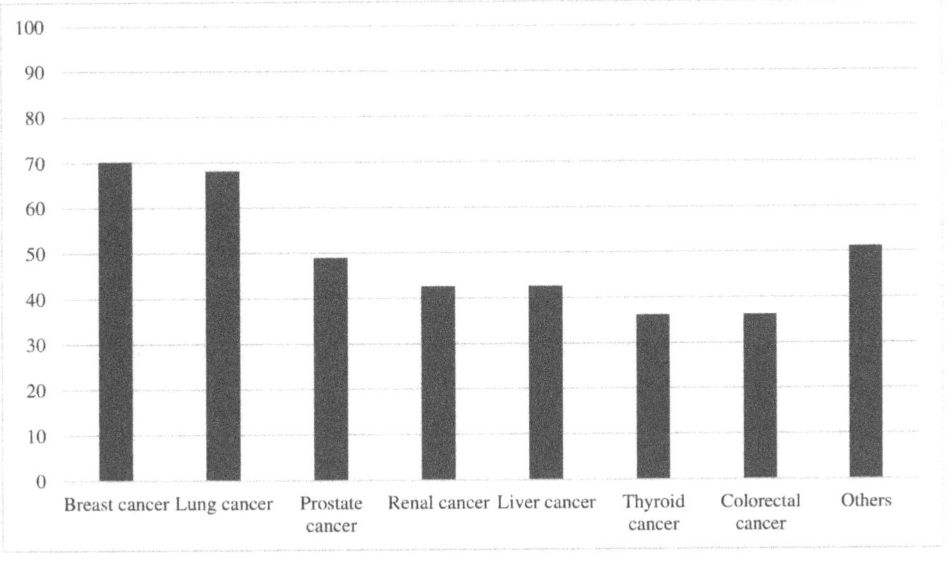

Figure 2. The percentage of how many studies feature specific primary tumor types is presented.

Table 3. AUC (training of each study's best model).

Study	Output/Prediction	Best-Performing Model	AUC	95% CI
Zhao et al. (2024) [6]	Hidden blood loss in spinal metastasis surgery	MRI-Based Radiomics	0.784	-
Bakhsheshian et al. (2022) [7]	Mortality	Machine Learning Model using ECI [1] and Frailty	0.788	-
	Medical complications		0.723	-
Massaad et al. (2022) [8]	1-year mortality	Machine Learning Model using Body Composition and NESMS [2]	0.73	0.67–0.78
Shi et al. (2022) [9]	Response of osteolytic metastases to chemotherapy	Radiomics (T2WI + ADC_{all})	0.908	0.86–0.96
Massaad et al. (2021) [10]	Postoperative complications	Random Forest to develop MSTFI [3]	0.62	0.56–0.68

The AUC and corresponding 95% confidence interval of studies reporting AUC values for the established radiomics models for the training of the model is presented. 1 = Elixhauser Comorbidity Index, 2 = New England Spinal Metastasis Score, 3 = Metastatic Spinal Tumor Frailty Index.

Table 4. AUC (internal validation of each study's best model).

Study	Output/Prediction	Best-Performing Model	AUC		95% CI	
Santipas et al. (2024) [11]	Complications after cervical spine metastases surgery	Gradient Boosting	0.939 [1]	0.873 [2]	-	-
Cui et al. (2024) [12]	Postoperative ambulatory status	Ensemble Machine Learning combining LR [6], eXGBM [7], SVM [8], RF [9], NN [10] and DT [11]	0.911 [1]		0.854–0.968 [1]	
Santipas et al. (2024) [13]	30-day preoperative VTE [5]	Gradient Boosted Trees	0.77 [1]		-	
	90-day preoperative VTE [5]	Support Vector Machine	0.72 [1]		-	
	30-day postoperative VTE [5]	Gradient Boosted Trees	0.71 [1]		-	
	90-day postoperative VTE [5]	Support Vector Machine	0.68 [1]		-	
Santipas et al. (2024) [14]	90-day survival	CatBoost	0.750 [1]	0.758 [2]	-	-
	180-day survival	XGBoost	0.726 [1]	0.744 [2]	-	-
	365-day survival	XGBoost	0.731 [1]	0.693 [2]	-	
Shi et al. (2024) [15]	Massive intraoperative blood loss	XGBoosting machine (XGBM; Machine Learning)	0.857 [2]		0.827–0.877 [2]	
Zhao et al. (2024) [6]	Hidden blood loss	MRI-Based Radiomics	0.744 [2]		0.576–0.914 [2]	
Chavalparit et al. (2023) [16]	90-day postoperative ambulatory status	Decision Tree	0.941 [1]		-	
	180-day postoperative ambulatory status	Extreme Gradient Boosting	0.852 [1]		-	
Chen et al. (2023) [17]	Treatment outcome after stereotactic body RT [12]	Gaussian Processes	0.828 [1]		-	
Gao et al. (2023) [18]	Severe psychological distress	Gradient Boosting Machine (Machine Learning)	0.865 [2]		0.788–0.941 [2]	
Hallinan et al. (2022) [19]	Grading metastatic epidural spinal cord compression (Bilsky grading (normal/low versus high)	Separated Window Learning (Max fusion model)	0.971 [2]		0.961–0.981 [2]	
	Grading metastatic epidural spinal cord compression (Bilsky grading (normal versus low/high)	Separated Window Learning (Spine-window)	0.924 [2]		0.910–0.938 [2]	
Jabehdar Maralani et al. (2022) [20]	Response following stereotactic body RT	Decision Tree	0.923 [1]	0.959 [2]	-	-
Karhade et al. (2022) [21]	6-week mortality	Elastic-net penalized logistic regression	0.85 [1]	0.84 [2]	0.84–0.86 [1]	0.80–0.88 [2]
Shi et al. (2022) [9]	Response of osteolytic metastases to chemotherapy	Radiomics (FST2WI + ADC_{all})	0.873 [2]		0.78–0.96 [2]	
Gui et al. (2022) [22]	Risk of vertebral compression fracture after stereotactic body RT [12]	Random Forest	0.878 [1]		0.832–0.924 [1]	
Massaad et al. (2021) [10]	Postoperative complications	Random Forest to develop MSTFI [3]	0.69 [4]		0.66–0.73 [4]	
Karhade et al. (2019) [23]	30-day mortality	Bayes Point Machine (Machine Learning)	0.786 [1]	0.782 [2]	-	-
Karhade et al. (2019) [24]	90-day mortality	Stochastic gradient boosting	0.83 [1]	0.83 [2]	0.81–0.85 [1]	-
	1-year mortality		0.85 [1]	0.89 [2]	0.83–0.87 [1]	-
Paulino Pereira et al. (2016) [25]	30-day survival	Boosting Algorithm; Nomogram	0.91 [1]	0.75 [2]	0.86–0.95 [1]	0.60–0.89 [2]
	90-day survival		0.86 [1]	0.73 [2]	0.83–0.90 [1]	0.63–0.83 [2]
	1-year survival		0.84 [1]	0.75 [2]	0.80–0.87 [1]	0.67–0.84 [2]

The AUC and corresponding 95% confidence interval of studies reporting AUC values for the established radiomics models for internal validation of the model is presented. 1 = k-fold cross validation, 2 = split sample internal validation, 3 = Metastatic Spinal Tumor Frailty Index, 4 = Internal Bootstrap Validation, 5 = venous thromboembolism, 6 = Logistic Regression, 7 = Extreme Gradient Boosting Machine, 8 = Support Vector Machine, 9 = Random Forest, 10 = Neural Network, 11 = Decision Tree, 12 = Radiotherapy.

Table 5. AUC (external validation of each study's best model).

Study	Output/Prediction	Best Performing Model	AUC	95% CI
Cui et al. (2024) [12]	Postoperative ambulatory status	Ensemble Machine Learning combining LR [2], eXGBM [3], SVM [4], RF [5], NN [6] and DT [7]	0.873	0.809–0.936
			0.924	0.890–0.959
Fenn et al. (2024) [26]	90-day mortality	Machine Learning Algorithm (SORG-MLA)	0.85	0.83–0.87
	1-year mortality		0.87	0.85–0.89
Huang et al. (2024) [27]	6-week survival	Machine Learning Algorithm (SORG-MLA)	0.84	0.78–0.89
	90-day survival		0.84	0.79–0.90
	1-year survival		0.77	0.73–0.80
Pan et al. (2024) [28]	42-day survival	Machine Learning Algorithm (SORG-MLA)	0.69	0.63–0.74
	90-day survival		0.72	0.66–0.77
	1-year survival		0.70	0.61–0.78
Shi et al. (2024) [15]	Massive intraoperative blood loss for spinal metastases	XGBoosting machine (XGBM; Machine Learning)	0.809	0.778–0.860
Li et al. (2023) [29]	90-day survival	Machine Learning Algorithm (SORG-MLA)	0.743	0.666–0.817
	180-day survival	Machine Learning Algorithm (Revised Katagiri)	0.761	0.696–0.826
	1-year survival	Machine Learning Algorithm (SORG-MLA)	0.787	0.730–0.838
	2-year survival	Machine Learning Algorithm (Revised Katagiri)	0.779	0.747–0.811
Su et al. (2023) [30]	6-week survival after RT [1] only	Machine Learning Algorithm (SORG-MLA)	0.77	0.74–0.79
	6-week survival after surgery		0.84	0.79–0.90
Zhong et al. (2023) [31]	90-day mortality	Machine Learning Algorithm (SORG-MLA)	0.714	0.589–0.839
	1-year mortality		0.832	0.758–0.906
Karhade et al. (2022) [21]	6-week mortality	Elastic-net penalized logistic regression	0.82	0.78–0.85
Yen et al. (2022) [32]	90-day survival	Machine Learning Algorithm (SORG-MLA)	0.78	0.76–0.80
	1-year survival		0.76	0.74–0.78
Shah et al. (2021) [33]	90-day mortality	Machine Learning Algorithm (SORG-MLA)	0.84	0.79–0.89
	1-year mortality		0.90	0.86–0.93
Yang et al. (2021) [34]	90-day mortality	Machine Learning Algorithm (SORG-MLA)	0.73	0.67–0.78
	1-year mortality		0.74	0.69–0.79
Bongers et al. (2020) [35]	90-day mortality	Machine Learning Algorithm (SORG-MLA)	0.81	0.74–0.87
	1-year mortality		0.84	0.77–0.89
Karhade et al. (2020) [36]	90-day mortality	Machine Learning Algorithm (SORG-MLA)	0.81	0.70–0.89
	1-year mortality		0.78	0.67–0.87

The AUC and corresponding 95% confidence interval of studies reporting AUC values for the established radiomics models for external validation of the model is presented. 1 = Radiation Therapy 2 = Logistic Regression, 3 = Extreme Gradient Boosting Machine, 4 = Support Vector Machine, 5 = Random Forest, 6 = Neural Network, 7 = Decision Tree.

The weighted average AUC value among the 18 studies that reported AUC values and corresponding 95% confidence intervals for internal validation of the established models is 0.876 (95% CI: 0.871–0.881). Wherever 95% confidence intervals were not reported, the weighted average of the reported 95% confidence intervals was used.

The weighted average AUC value among the eight studies that reported AUC values and corresponding 95% confidence intervals for external validation of the established models is 0.810 (95% CI: 0.803–0.816).

Meta-Analysis of the SORG-MLA Model

The pooled AUC of the SORG-MLA model for 90-day survival was 0.79 (95% CI: 0.75–0.82) and for 1-year survival 0.80 (95% CI: 0.75–0.85). The prediction intervals ranged from 0.65 to 0.88 and from 0.62 to 0.91, respectively. Figures 3 and 4 are forest plots of the 90-day survival and 1-year survival.

4. Discussion

The integration of artificial intelligence (AI) into clinical oncology is revolutionizing the care of patients with spinal metastases. Here, data were combined from 47 studies with a pool of >25,000 patients with a range of models presented for a breadth of clinical applications, from predicting surgical mortality and complications to estimating occult blood loss and assessing perioperative functional status. The heterogeneity of use-cases highlights the versatility of AI for addressing different facets of managing spinal metastases. Notably, prediction models demonstrated strong discriminative performance with pooled AUC values of 0.762, 0.876, and 0.810 for training, internal, and external validation, respectively, supporting the reasonable accuracy and generalizability of these models across multiple datasets (Tables 3–5). Additionally, the predominance of certain primary tumor types, including breast, lung, and prostate, within the included studies reflects their real-world contribution to spinal metastases. While this focus ensures relevance to a large patient population, it also raises questions about generalizability of these models to rarer malignancies which might be underrepresented, including neuroendocrine or esophageal sources. There is a need for more balanced datasets and the inclusion of between- and within-subgroup analyses to account for tumor-type-specific variability in outcomes and treatment response.

Reproducibility remains a fundamental challenge in radiomics-based models due to variability in image acquisition protocols, reconstruction parameters, and scanner types across institutions. These inconsistencies can substantially alter extracted radiomic features, thereby affecting model performance when applied outside the development cohort [37]. Our review noted that only a minority of studies implemented harmonization techniques such as image resampling, intensity normalization, or ComBat-based feature adjustment, which aim to mitigate site-specific variability. The lack of standardization across studies limits generalizability and may contribute to overfitting or unstable performance in external validation cohorts [37]. Future research should prioritize standardized radiomics pipelines and transparent reporting of acquisition parameters to enable reliable replication and multi-center deployment of radiomics-based predictive tools.

Crucially, survival prediction emerged as the most extensively studied application of AI in spinal metastasis, with several model algorithms, especially those developed by the Skeletal Oncology Research Group (SORG), subject to both internal and international external validation. The consistent performance of these models across different populations and healthcare infrastructures supports their utility as decision-support tools [23,24,30,33]. For instance, models predicting 90-day and 1-year mortality yielded AUCs approaching or exceeding 0.84 in many studies, making a strong case for these tools to be used in preoperative planning or when evaluating eligibility for aggressive intervention [21,23,24,35,36]. Despite this, all studies that externally evaluated the SORG-MLA were retrospective in their design, thereby limiting the real-world significance of the pooled AUCs. Therefore, the realization of real-world impact studies is encouraged to assess clinical endpoints such as changes in treatment decisions and improved survival.

Although AI models' prognostic abilities in spinal metastases have shown promise, the discipline is still struggling with the crucial problems of interpretability and explainability. The safe and moral incorporation of AI into healthcare decision-making depends on these factors. The fact that many of the evaluated research rely on opaque, sophisticated algorithms, including deep neural networks and ensemble-based models like XGBoost, random forest, CatBoost, or Gaussian processes, without providing clear reasoning routes, is a major drawback [12,13,15,17,18,20,21]. A model must be interpretable in order to promote patient acceptance, clinician trust, and regulatory compliance in the therapeutic setting, where decisions have significant consequences [3,10].

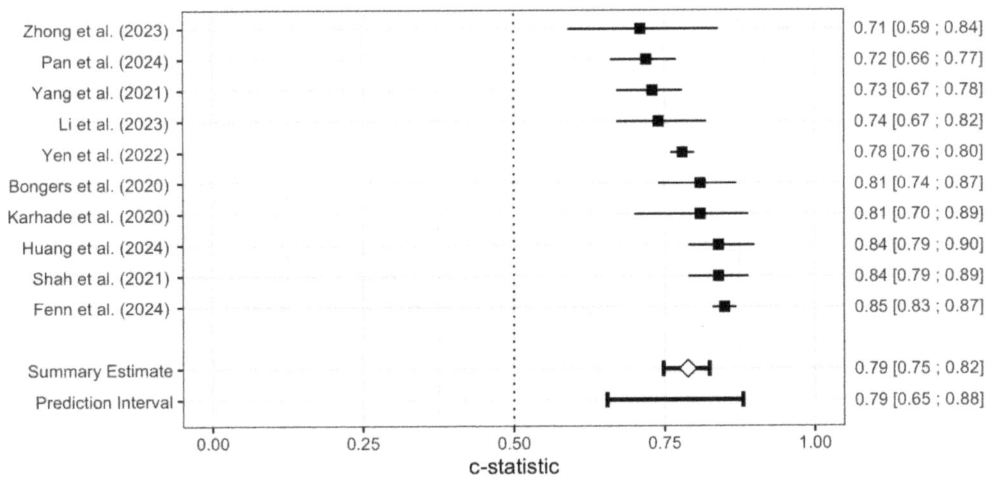

Figure 3. A Forest plot of the meta-analysis of the AUC for the SORG-MLA model for 90-day survival is shown. The AUC and 95% Confidence Intervals of each independent model validation are depicted. The diamond represents the pooled AUC along with a 95% Confidence Interval. A prediction interval is presented [26–29,31–36].

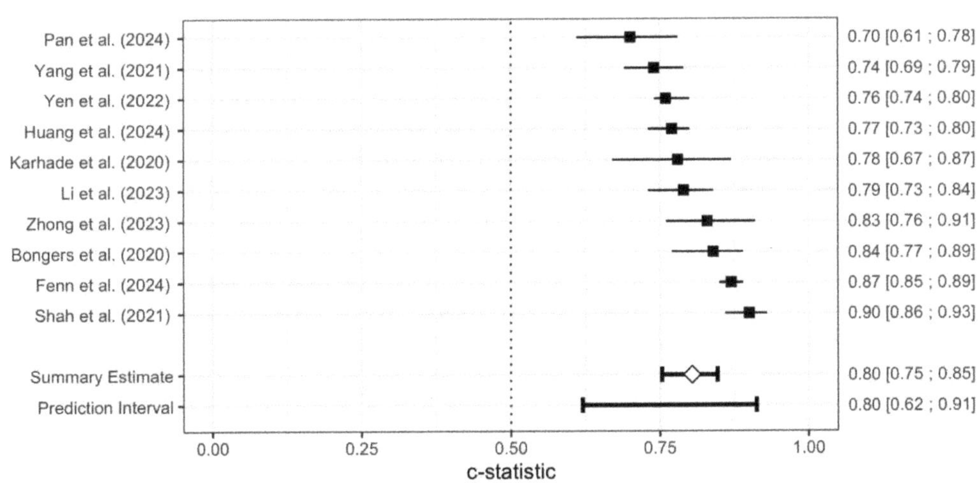

Figure 4. Forest plot of the meta-analysis of the AUC for the SORG-MLA model for 1-year survival. The AUC and 95% Confidence Intervals of each independent model validation are depicted. The diamond represents the pooled AUC along with a 95% Confidence Interval. A prediction interval is presented [26–29,31–36].

Because it is difficult to understand how input features affect predictions, there is rising worry that "black box" models might be dangerous for patient care [10,15,17]. However, only a small percentage of the papers we examined used explainable AI (XAI) methods to help physicians and stakeholders understand the model's logic, such as SHAP (Shapley Additive Explanations), LIME (Local Interpretable Model-Agnostic Explanations), or decision-path visualizations. For example, there was little investigation into the methods by which high-performing models created with random forest [10,22], support vector machines [13], and deep learning [19] arrived at their predictions.

Adoption in multidisciplinary decision-making settings [5], when physicians are held responsible for defending treatment decisions, may be constrained by this lack of openness. It will be crucial to include model interpretability tools (such as attention heatmaps and feature significance plots) into upcoming development workflows. AI in spine cancer cannot be meaningfully implemented without clinician-centered design, explainable model architecture, and cross-validation across a variety of datasets [3,25].

Adoption and clinical implementation of AI models is largely dependent on the ease of use and availability of such models. We identified six studies [12,15,21,23,24,27] that deployed a user-friendly platform, i.e., web-based applications. Of these studies, only two web-based applications [21,24] were working trouble-free at the time of the creation of this manuscript. The two functioning applications represent the SORG-MLA at different time points, which have been integrated into one website [24]. Such availability builds the foundation on which clinical uptake and regular usage is dependent. Therefore, more models should be made readily available by deploying them via user-friendly platforms, such as websites, mobile apps etc.

5. Limitations

We have now added a specific Limitations Section to offer a thorough and open evaluation of the limitations of this research. Regarding data preparation, outcome definitions, validation methods, and reporting standards, the included studies exhibit methodological variability. To reduce direct cross-comparability of model performance, for example, some research used split-sample validation or no validation at all, while others used k-fold cross-validation [14,15,21].

Second, there is significant worry about demographic and regional bias across datasets. The bulk of training cohorts come from middle- to high-income nations like China, Taiwan, and the United States [21,30,31,34], which can restrict the applicability of AI tools to underrepresented groups or environments with limited resources. International external validation studies are available [31,33,34], but few of them specifically address equality, cultural adaptability, or the diversity of healthcare systems when using AI. Further external validation should thus be carried out to ensure applicability and global generalizability of existing models. Ethnic or racial biases are addressed in some studies; however, the homogenous nature of many validation cohorts does not allow for adequate distinctions of model performance between different ethnic or racial groups to be made. Future models should therefore be trained on a heterogenous pool of patients to account for cultural, ethnic, racial, and socioeconomic differences.

Third, while some models showed good discrimination metrics (AUCs > 0.85), we were unable to fully evaluate the clinical value of these tools since calibration metrics and decision-curve analysis were seldom published [23,25,32]. It is noteworthy that the majority of models are still in the research realm and have not yet been included into real-time clinical decision processes or electronic health records (EHRs2). The limited number of studies that documented attempts to create web-based apps or clinician-facing tools [15,38] limited its translational preparedness.

Lastly, the examined literature still lacks sufficient attention to ethical and practical concerns, such as patient privacy, data completeness, interpretability, and openness. For instance, in several studies, missing variables (such as albumin or lymphocyte counts) deteriorated model performance [27], but few models included flexible topologies or robust imputation to deal with such uncertainty. Future multicenter, prospective, inclusive studies that assess the practical performance, equity, and stakeholder acceptance of AI tools in spinal cancer are desperately needed, as these data highlight.

6. Conclusions

AI has the potential to advance spinal metastasis care in the domains of outcome prediction and risk stratification and thus enhance precision medicine and streamline clinical workflow to improve patient outcomes. If rigorously validated and ethically deployed, AI has the potential not just to predict outcomes but to transform spinal oncology into a more personalized, equitable, and data-driven discipline. As AI continues to evolve within spinal oncology, its success will depend not only on predictive accuracy but also on transparency, interpretability, and ethical deployment. Future models must prioritize explainability to foster clinician trust, support informed consent, and ensure equitable care across diverse patient populations.

Supplementary Materials: The following supporting information can be downloaded at: https://www.mdpi.com/article/10.3390/jcm14165885/s1, Supplementary Figure S1: Risk of bias. Supplementary Figure S2: Applicability. Supplementary Table S1: Search queries across databases. Supplementary Table S2: Summary of the studies analyzed. References [39–53] are cited in the supplementary materials.

Author Contributions: Conceptualization, V.S.; Methodology, V.S.; Formal Analysis, V.S. and A.T.; Investigation, V.S., P.D., Z.L. and P.H.; Data Curation, V.S., P.D.; Writing—Original Draft Preparation, V.S.; Writing—Review and Editing, V.S., P.D., A.T., Z.L., P.H., S.H., E.O.R.N., M.J.C., J.R. and A.D.; Supervision, J.R. and A.D.; Project Administration, vs. All authors have read and agreed to the published version of the manuscript.

Funding: This research received no external funding.

Institutional Review Board Statement: Ethical review and approval were waived for this study due it being a systematic review of previously published data and did not involve human participants or the collection of new data.

Data Availability Statement: All datasets used for this study are presented in the manuscript and its Supplementary Materials.

Conflicts of Interest: The authors declare no conflicts of interest.

References

1. Wewel, J.T.; O'Toole, J.E. Epidemiology of spinal cord and column tumors. *Neuro-Oncol. Pract.* **2020**, *7* (Suppl. S1), i5–i9. [CrossRef]
2. Conti, A.; Acker, G.; Kluge, A.; Loebel, F.; Kreimeier, A.; Budach, V.; Vajkoczy, P.; Ghetti, I.; Germano', A.F.; Senger, C.; et al. Decision Making in Patients with Metastatic Spine. The Role of Minimally Invasive Treatment Modalities. *Front. Oncol.* **2019**, *9*, 915. [CrossRef]
3. Dixon, D.; Sattar, H.; Moros, N.; Kesireddy, S.R.; Ahsan, H.; Lakkimsetti, M.; Fatima, M.; Doshi, D.; Sadhu, K.; Junaid Hassan, M. Unveiling the Influence of AI Predictive Analytics on Patient Outcomes: A Comprehensive Narrative Review. *Cureus* **2024**, *16*, e59954. [CrossRef]
4. Barton, L.B.; Arant, K.R.; Blucher, J.A.; Sarno, D.L.; Redmond, K.J.; Balboni, T.A.; Colman, M.; Goodwin, C.R.; Laufer, I.; Placide, R.; et al. Clinician Experiences in Treatment Decision-Making for Patients with Spinal Metastases. *J. Bone Jt. Surg.* **2021**, *103*, e1. [CrossRef] [PubMed]
5. Sanker, V.; Sanikommu, S.; Thaller, A.; Li, Z.; Heesen, P.; Hariharan, S.; Nordin, E.O.R.; Cavagnaro, M.J.; Ratliff, J.; Desai, A. Artificial Intelligence for Non-Invasive Prediction of Molecular Signatures in Spinal Metastases: A Systematic Review. *Bioengineering* **2025**, *12*, 791. [CrossRef]
6. Zhao, W.; Qin, S.; Wang, Q.; Chen, Y.; Liu, K.; Xin, P.; Lang, N. Assessment of Hidden Blood Loss in Spinal Metastasis Surgery: A Comprehensive Approach with MRI-Based Radiomics Models. *J. Magn. Reson. Imaging* **2024**, *59*, 2023–2032. [CrossRef] [PubMed]
7. Bakhsheshian, J.; Shahrestani, S.; Buser, Z.; Hah, R.; Hsieh, P.C.; Liu, J.C.; Wang, J.C. The performance of frailty in predictive modeling of short-term outcomes in the surgical management of metastatic tumors to the spine. *Spine J.* **2022**, *22*, 605–615. [CrossRef]

8. Massaad, E.; Bridge, C.P.; Kiapour, A.; Fourman, M.S.; Duvall, J.B.; Connolly, I.D.; Hadzipasic, M.; Shankar, G.M.; Andriole, K.P.; Rosenthal, M.; et al. Evaluating frailty, mortality, and complications associated with metastatic spine tumor surgery using machine learning–derived body composition analysis. *J. Neurosurg. Spine* **2022**, *37*, 263–273. [CrossRef]
9. Shi, Y.J.; Zhu, H.T.; Li, X.T.; Zhang, X.Y.; Wei, Y.Y.; Yan, S.; Sun, Y.S. Radiomics analysis based on multiple parameters MR imaging in the spine: Predicting treatment response of osteolytic bone metastases to chemotherapy in breast cancer patients. *Magn. Reson. Imaging* **2022**, *92*, 10–18. [CrossRef]
10. Massaad, E.; Williams, N.; Hadzipasic, M.; Patel, S.S.; Fourman, M.S.; Kiapour, A.; Schoenfeld, A.J.; Shankar, G.M.; Shin, J.H. Performance assessment of the metastatic spinal tumor frailty index using machine learning algorithms: Limitations and future directions. *Neurosurg. Focus* **2021**, *50*, E5. [CrossRef]
11. Santipas, B.; Suvithayasiri, S.; Trathitephun, W.; Wilartratsami, S.; Luksanapruksa, P. Developmental and Validation of Machine Learning Model for Prediction Complication After Cervical Spine Metastases Surgery. *Clin. Spine Surgery: A Spine Publ.* **2024**, *38*, E81–E88. [CrossRef]
12. Cui, Y.; Shi, X.; Qin, Y.; Wang, Q.; Cao, X.; Che, X.; Pan, Y.; Wang, B.; Lei, M.; Liu, Y. Establishment and validation of an interactive artificial intelligence platform to predict postoperative ambulatory status for patients with metastatic spinal disease: A multicenter analysis. *Int. J. Surg.* **2024**, *110*, 2738–2756. [CrossRef]
13. Santipas, B.; Chanajit, A.; Wilartratsami, S.; Ittichaiwong, P.; Veerakanjana, K.; Luksanapruksa, P. Development of Machine Learning Algorithms for Predicting Preoperative and Postoperative venous Thromboembolism in Patients Undergoing Surgery for Spinal Metastasis. *Siriraj Med. J.* **2024**, *76*, 381–388. [CrossRef]
14. Santipas, B.; Veerakanjana, K.; Ittichaiwong, P.; Chavalparit, P.; Wilartratsami, S.; Luksanapruksa, P. Development and internal validation of machine-learning models for predicting survival in patients who underwent surgery for spinal metastases. *Asian Spine J.* **2024**, *18*, 325–335. [CrossRef]
15. Shi, X.; Cui, Y.; Wang, S.; Pan, Y.; Wang, B.; Lei, M. Development and validation of a web-based artificial intelligence prediction model to assess massive intraoperative blood loss for metastatic spinal disease using machine learning techniques. *Spine J.* **2024**, *24*, 146–160. [CrossRef] [PubMed]
16. Chavalparit, P.; Wilartratsami, S.; Santipas, B.; Ittichaiwong, P.; Veerakanjana, K.; Luksanapruksa, P. Development of Machine-Learning Models to Predict Ambulation Outcomes Following Spinal Metastasis Surgery. *Asian Spine J.* **2023**, *17*, 1013–1023. [CrossRef] [PubMed]
17. Chen, Y.; Qin, S.; Zhao, W.; Wang, Q.; Liu, K.; Xin, P.; Yuan, H.; Zhuang, H.; Lang, N. MRI feature-based radiomics models to predict treatment outcome after stereotactic body radiotherapy for spinal metastases. *Insights Into Imaging* **2023**, *14*, 169. [CrossRef] [PubMed]
18. Gao, L.; Cao, Y.; Cao, X.; Shi, X.; Lei, M.; Su, X.; Liu, Y. Machine learning-based algorithms to predict severe psychological distress among cancer patients with spinal metastatic disease. *Spine J.* **2023**, *23*, 1255–1269. [CrossRef]
19. Hallinan, J.T.P.D.; Zhu, L.; Zhang, W.; Kuah, T.; Lim, D.S.W.; Low, X.Z.; Cheng, A.J.L.; Eide, S.E.; Ong, H.Y.; Muhamat Nor, F.E.; et al. Deep Learning Model for Grading Metastatic Epidural Spinal Cord Compression on Staging CT. *Cancers* **2022**, *14*, 3219. [CrossRef]
20. Jabehdar Maralani, P.; Chen, H.; Moazen, B.; Mojtahed Zadeh, M.; Salehi, F.; Chan, A.; Zeng, L.K.; Abugharib, A.; Tseng, C.L.; Husain, Z.; et al. Proposing a quantitative MRI-based linear measurement framework for response assessment following stereotactic body radiation therapy in patients with spinal metastasis. *J. Neurooncol.* **2022**, *160*, 265–272. [CrossRef]
21. Karhade, A.V.; Fenn, B.; Groot, O.Q.; Shah, A.A.; Yen, H.K.; Bilsky, M.H.; Hu, M.H.; Laufer, I.; Park, D.Y.; Sciubba, D.M.; et al. Development and external validation of predictive algorithms for six-week mortality in spinal metastasis using 4304 patients from five institutions. *Spine J.* **2022**, *22*, 2033–2041. [CrossRef]
22. Gui, C.; Chen, X.; Sheikh, K.; Mathews, L.; Lo, S.L.; Lee, J.; Khan, M.A.; Sciubba, D.M.; Redmond, K.J. Radiomic modeling to predict risk of vertebral compression fracture after stereotactic body radiation therapy for spinal metastases. *J. Neurosurg. Spine* **2022**, *36*, 294–302. [CrossRef]
23. Karhade, A.V.; Thio, Q.C.B.S.; Ogink, P.T.; Shah, A.A.; Bono, C.M.; Oh, K.S.; Saylor, P.J.; Schoenfeld, A.J.; Shin, J.H.; Harris, M.B.; et al. Development of Machine Learning Algorithms for Prediction of 30-Day Mortality After Surgery for Spinal Metastasis. *Neurosurgery* **2019**, *85*, E83–E91. [CrossRef]
24. Karhade, A.V.; Thio, Q.C.B.S.; Ogink, P.T.; Bono, C.M.; Ferrone, M.L.; Oh, K.S.; Saylor, P.J.; Schoenfeld, A.J.; Shin, J.H.; Harris, M.B.; et al. Predicting 90-Day and 1-Year Mortality in Spinal Metastatic Disease: Development and Internal Validation. *Neurosurgery* **2019**, *85*, E671–E681. [CrossRef]
25. Paulino Pereira, N.R.; Janssen, S.J.; van Dijk, E.; Harris, M.B.; Hornicek, F.J.; Ferrone, M.L.; Schwab, J.H. Development of a Prognostic Survival Algorithm for Patients with Metastatic Spine Disease. *J. Bone Jt. Surg.* **2016**, *98*, 1767–1776. [CrossRef] [PubMed]

26. Fenn, B.P.; Karhade, A.V.; Groot, O.Q.; Collins, A.K.; Balboni, T.A.; Oh, K.S.; Ferrone, M.L.; Schwab, J.H. Survival in Patients with Spinal Metastatic Disease Treated Nonoperatively with Radiotherapy. *Clin. Spine Surgery A Spine Publ.* **2024**, *37*, E290–E296. [CrossRef] [PubMed]
27. Huang, C.C.; Peng, K.P.; Hsieh, H.C.; Groot, O.Q.; Yen, H.K.; Tsai, C.C.; Karhade, A.V.; Lin, Y.P.; Kao, Y.T.; Yang, J.J.; et al. Does the Presence of Missing Data Affect the Performance of the SORG Machine-learning Algorithm for Patients with Spinal Metastasis? Development of an Internet Application Algorithm. *Clin. Orthop. Relat. Res.* **2024**, *482*, 143–157. [CrossRef] [PubMed]
28. Pan, Y.T.; Lin, Y.P.; Yen, H.K.; Yen, H.H.; Huang, C.C.; Hsieh, H.C.; Janssen, S.; Hu, M.H.; Lin, W.H.; Groot, O.Q. Are Current Survival Prediction Tools Useful When Treating Subsequent Skeletal-related Events From Bone Metastases? *Clin. Orthop. Relat. Res.* **2024**, *482*, 1710–1721. [CrossRef] [PubMed]
29. Li, Z.; Guo, L.; Guo, B.; Zhang, P.; Wang, J.; Wang, X.; Yao, W. Evaluation of different scoring systems for spinal metastases based on a Chinese cohort. *Cancer Med.* **2023**, *12*, 4125–4136. [CrossRef]
30. Su, C.C.; Lin, Y.P.; Yen, H.K.; Pan, Y.T.; Zijlstra, H.; Verlaan, J.J.; Schwab, J.H.; Lai, C.Y.; Hu, M.H.; Yang, S.H.; et al. A Machine Learning Algorithm for Predicting 6-Week Survival in Spinal Metastasis: An External Validation Study Using 2768 Taiwanese Patients. *J. Am. Acad. Orthop. Surg.* **2023**, *31*, e645–e656. [CrossRef]
31. Zhong, G.; Cheng, S.; Zhou, M.; Xie, J.; Xu, Z.; Lai, H.; Yan, Y.; Xie, Z.; Zhou, J.; Xie, X.; et al. External validation of the SORG machine learning algorithms for predicting 90-day and 1-year survival of patients with lung cancer-derived spine metastases: A recent bi-center cohort from China. *Spine J.* **2023**, *23*, 731–738. [CrossRef]
32. Yen, H.K.; Hu, M.H.; Zijlstra, H.; Groot, O.Q.; Hsieh, H.C.; Yang, J.J.; Karhade, A.V.; Chen, P.C.; Chen, Y.H.; Huang, P.H.; et al. Prognostic significance of lab data and performance comparison by validating survival prediction models for patients with spinal metastases after radiotherapy. *Radiother. Oncol.* **2022**, *175*, 159–166. [CrossRef] [PubMed]
33. Shah, A.A.; Karhade, A.V.; Park, H.Y.; Sheppard, W.L.; Macyszyn, L.J.; Everson, R.G.; Shamie, A.N.; Park, D.Y.; Schwab, J.H.; Hornicek, F.J. Updated external validation of the SORG machine learning algorithms for prediction of ninety-day and one-year mortality after surgery for spinal metastasis. *Spine J.* **2021**, *21*, 1679–1686. [CrossRef] [PubMed]
34. Yang, J.J.; Chen, C.W.; Fourman, M.S.; Bongers, M.E.R.; Karhade, A.V.; Groot, O.Q.; Lin, W.H.; Yen, H.K.; Huang, P.H.; Yang, S.H.; et al. International external validation of the SORG machine learning algorithms for predicting 90-day and one-year survival of patients with spine metastases using a Taiwanese cohort. *Spine J.* **2021**, *21*, 1670–1678. [CrossRef]
35. Bongers, M.E.R.; Karhade, A.V.; Villavieja, J.; Groot, O.Q.; Bilsky, M.H.; Laufer, I.; Schwab, J.H. Does the SORG algorithm generalize to a contemporary cohort of patients with spinal metastases on external validation? *Spine J.* **2020**, *20*, 1646–1652. [CrossRef]
36. Karhade, A.V.; Ahmed, A.K.; Pennington, Z.; Chara, A.; Schilling, A.; Thio, Q.C.B.S.; Ogink, P.T.; Sciubba, D.M.; Schwab, J.H. External validation of the SORG 90-day and 1-year machine learning algorithms for survival in spinal metastatic disease. *Spine J.* **2020**, *20*, 14–21. [CrossRef]
37. Lee, S.B.; Hong, Y.; Cho, Y.J.; Jeong, D.; Lee, J.; Choi, J.W.; Hwang, J.Y.; Lee, S.; Choi, Y.H.; Cheon, J.E. Enhancing Radiomics Reproducibility: Deep Learning-Based Harmonization of Abdominal Computed Tomography (CT) Images. *Bioengineering* **2024**, *11*, 1212. [CrossRef]
38. He, X.; Jiao, Y.Q.; Yang, X.G.; Hu, Y.C. A Novel Prediction Tool for Overall Survival of Patients Living with Spinal Metastatic Disease. *World Neurosurg.* **2020**, *144*, e824–e836. [CrossRef]
39. Kehayias, C.E.; Bontempi, D.; Quirk, S.; Friesen, S.; Bredfeldt, J.; Kosak, T.; Kearney, M.; Tishler, R.; Pashtan, I.; Huynh, M.A.; et al. A prospectively deployed deep learning-enabled automated quality assurance tool for oncological palliative spine radiation therapy. *Lancet Digit. Health* **2024**, *7*, e13–e22. [CrossRef]
40. Li, J.; Zhang, J.; Zhang, X.; Lun, D.; Li, R.; Ma, R.; Hu, Y. Quantile regression-based prediction of intraoperative blood loss in patients with spinal metastases: Model development and validation. *Eur. Spine J.* **2023**, *32*, 2479–2492. [CrossRef]
41. Mezei, T.; Horváth, A.; Nagy, Z.; Czigléczki, G.; Banczerowski, P.; Báskay, J.; Pollner, P. A Novel Prognostication System for Spinal Metastasis Patients Based on Network Science and Correlation Analysis. *Clin. Oncol.* **2022**, *35*, e20–e29. [CrossRef]
42. Fourman, M.S.; Siraj, L.; Duvall, J.; Ramsey, D.C.; De La Garza Ramos, R.; Hadzipasic, M.; Connolly, I.; Williamson, T.; Shankar, G.M.; Schoenfeld, A.; et al. Can We Use Artificial Intelligence Cluster Analysis to Identify Patients with Metastatic Breast Cancer to the Spine at Highest Risk of Postoperative Adverse Events? *World Neurosurg.* **2023**, *174*, e26–e34. [CrossRef]
43. Li, Z.; Huang, L.; Guo, B.; Zhang, P.; Wang, J.; Wang, X.; Yao, W. The predictive ability of routinely collected laboratory markers for surgically treated spinal metastases: A retrospective single institution study. BMC Cancer. *MC Cancer* **2022**, *22*, 1231. [CrossRef]
44. Hu, M.H.; Yen, H.K.; Chen, I.H.; Wu, C.H.; Chen, C.W.; Yang, J.J.; Wang, Z.Y.; Yen, M.H.; Yang, S.H.; Lin, W.H. Decreased psoas muscle area is a prognosticator for 90-day and 1-year survival in patients undergoing surgical treatment for spinal metastasis. *Clin. Nutr.* **2022**, *41*, 620–629. [CrossRef]
45. Walker, A.; Bassale, S.; Shukla, R.; Dai Kubicky, C. A Prognostic Index for Predicting Survival of Patients Undergoing Radiation Therapy for Spine Metastasis Using Recursive Partitioning Analysis. *J. Palliat. Med.* **2022**, *25*, 21–27. [CrossRef]

46. Khalid, S.I.; Massaad, E.; Kiapour, A.; Bridge, C.P.; Rigney, G.; Burrows, A.; Shim, J.; De la Garza Ramos, R.; Tobert, D.G.; Schoenfeld, A.J.; et al. Machine learning–based detection of sarcopenic obesity and association with adverse outcomes in patients undergoing surgical treatment for spinal metastases. *J. Neurosurg. Spine* **2024**, *40*, 291–300. [CrossRef] [PubMed]
47. Rigney, G.H.; Massaad, E.; Kiapour, A.; Razak, S.S.; Duvall, J.B.; Burrows, A.; Khalid, S.I.; De La Garza Ramos, R.; Tobert, D.G.; Williamson, T.; et al. Implication of nutritional status for adverse outcomes after surgery for metastatic spine tumors. *J. Neurosurg. Spine* **2023**, *39*, 557–567. [CrossRef] [PubMed]
48. Hallinan, J.T.P.D.; Zhu, L.; Zhang, W.; Lim, D.S.W.; Baskar, S.; Low, X.Z.; Yeong, K.Y.; Teo, E.C.; Kumarakulasinghe, N.B.; Yap, Q.V.; et al. Deep Learning Model for Classifying Metastatic Epidural Spinal Cord Compression on MRI. *Front. Oncol.* **2022**, *12*, 849447. [CrossRef] [PubMed]
49. Arends, S.R.S.; Savenije, M.H.F.; Eppinga, W.S.C.; van der Velden, J.M.; van den Berg, C.A.T.; Verhoeff, J.J.C. Clinical utility of convolutional neural networks for treatment planning in radiotherapy for spinal metastases. *Phys. Imaging Radiat. Oncol.* **2022**, *21*, 42–47. [CrossRef]
50. Rogé, M.; Henni, A.H.; Neggaz, Y.A.; Mallet, R.; Hanzen, C.; Dubray, B.; Colard, E.; Gensanne, D.; Thureau, S. Evaluation of a Dedicated Software "Elements^{TM} Spine SRS, Brainlab$^{®}$" for Target Volume Definition in the Treatment of Spinal Bone Metastases with Stereotactic Body Radiotherapy. *Front Oncol.* **2022**, *12*, 827195. [CrossRef]
51. Kowalchuk, R.O.; Waters, M.R.; Richardson, K.M.; Spencer, K.; Larner, J.M.; McAllister, W.H.; Sheehan, J.P.; Kersh, C.R. Stereotactic body radiation therapy for spinal metastases: A novel local control stratification by spinal region. *J. Neurosurg. Spine* **2021**, *34*, 267–276. [CrossRef]
52. Korpics, M.C.; Polley, M.Y.; Bhave, S.R.; Redler, G.; Pitroda, S.P.; Luke, J.J.; Chmura, S.J. A Validated T Cell Radiomics Score Is Associated with Clinical Outcomes Following Multisite SBRT and Pembrolizumab. *Int. J. Radiat. Oncol. Biol. Phys.* **2020**, *108*, 189–195. [CrossRef]
53. Cui, Y.; Pan, Y.; Lei, M.; Mi, C.; Wang, B.; Shi, X. The First Algorithm Calculating Cement Injection Volumes in Patients with Spine Metastases Treated with Percutaneous Vertebroplasty. *Ther. Clin. Risk Manag.* **2020**, *16*, 417–4288. [CrossRef]

Journal of
Clinical Medicine

MDPI

Systematic Review

Applications and Performance of Artificial Intelligence in Spinal Metastasis Imaging: A Systematic Review

Vivek Sanker [1,*], Poorvikha Gowda [2], Alexander Thaller [3], Zhikai Li [4], Philip Heesen [5], Zekai Qiang [6], Srinath Hariharan [1], Emil O. R. Nordin [1], Maria Jose Cavagnaro [1], John Ratliff [1] and Atman Desai [1]

1 Department of Neurosurgery, Stanford University, Palo Alto, CA 94305, USA; hsrinath@stanford.edu (S.H.); enordin@stanford.edu (E.O.R.N.); mjcava@stanford.edu (M.J.C.); jratliff@stanford.edu (J.R.); atman@stanford.edu (A.D.)
2 Department of Neurosurgery, St John's Medical College, Bangalore 560034, Karnataka, India; poorvikha2712@gmail.com
3 Department of Neurosurgery, Medical University of Graz, 8010 Graz, Styria, Austria; alexander.thaller@medunigraz.at
4 Department of Clinical Neurosciences, Addenbrooke's Hospital, Cambridge CB2 0QQ, UK; zl498@cam.ac.uk
5 Faculty of Medicine, University of Zurich, 8032 Zurich, Switzerland; heesenphilip99@gmail.com
6 School of Medicine and Population Health, University of Sheffield Medical School, Sheffield S10 2RX, UK
* Correspondence: vsanker@stanford.edu

Abstract: Background: Spinal metastasis is the third most common site for metastatic localization, following the lung and liver. Manual detection through imaging modalities such as CT, MRI, PET, and bone scintigraphy can be costly and inefficient. Preliminary artificial intelligence (AI) techniques and computer-aided detection (CAD) systems have attempted to improve lesion detection, segmentation, and treatment response in oncological imaging. The objective of this review is to evaluate the current applications of AI across multimodal imaging techniques in the diagnosis of spinal metastasis. **Methods:** Databases like PubMed, Scopus, Web of Science Advance, Cochrane, and Embase (Ovid) were searched using specific keywords like 'spine metastases', 'artificial intelligence', 'machine learning', 'deep learning', and 'diagnosis'. The screening of studies adhered to the PRISMA guidelines. Relevant variables were extracted from each of the included articles such as the primary tumor type, cohort size, and prediction model performance metrics: area under the receiver operating curve (AUC), accuracy, sensitivity, specificity, internal validation and external validation. A random-effects meta-analysis model was used to account for variability between the studies. Quality assessment was performed using the PROBAST tool. **Results:** This review included 39 studies published between 2007 and 2024, encompassing a total of 6267 patients. The three most common primary tumors were lung cancer (56.4%), breast cancer (51.3%), and prostate cancer (41.0%). Four studies reported AUC values for model training, 16 for internal validation, and five for external validation. The weighted average AUCs were 0.971 (training), 0.947 (internal validation), and 0.819 (external validation). The risk of bias was the highest in the analysis domain, with 22 studies (56%) rated high risk, primarily due to inadequate external validation and overfitting. **Conclusions:** AI-based approaches show promise for enhancing the detection, segmentation, and characterization of spinal metastatic lesions across multiple imaging modalities. Future research should focus on developing more generalizable models through larger and more diverse training datasets, integrating clinical and imaging data, and conducting prospective validation studies to demonstrate meaningful clinical impact.

Keywords: artificial intelligence (AI); spinal metastasis; diagnostic imaging; deep learning; convolutional neural networks (CNNs); radiomics; machine learning

 https://doi.org/10.3390/jcm14165877

1. Introduction

Spinal metastasis represents the third most common site for metastatic localization, following the lung and the liver [1]. Nearly 70% of the primary breast and prostate tumors are metastasized to the axial skeleton due to its high red marrow content which can in turn lead to a spectrum of clinical manifestations and immensely impact a patient's quality of life. Complications include pathological fractures, spinal cord compression, spinal deformity, and reduced mobility and neurological deficits, which can progress and be irreversible without early treatment [2]. Therefore, early detection and diagnosis play a pivotal role in clinical practice [3]. Advanced imaging techniques such as computed tomography (CT), magnetic resonance imaging (MRI), positron emission tomography (PET), and bone scintigraphy are typically used in assessing osseous metastases. The sensitivity and specificity of CT, MRI, PET and bone scintigraphy are reported to be 79.2% and 92.3%, 94.1% and 94.2%, 89.8% and 63.3%, and 80.0% and 92.8%, respectively [4].

The detection of spinal metastasis through these various imaging modalities is often time-consuming and challenging. Recently, preliminary artificial intelligence (AI) techniques and computer-aided detection (CAD) software systems have been applied in medical imaging applications, particularly in oncological imaging [5]. The use of machine learning techniques such as radiomics-based feature analysis and convolutional neural networks (CNNs) have been studied for lesion detection, segmentation, and treatment response [6]. Radiomics, in principle, is capable of extracting subtle features from images beyond those inferable to the human eye, but one disadvantage is that it requires the extraction of handcrafted features [7]; however, this can potentially be circumvented by employing deep learning techniques which learn important imaging features for classification through a hierarchical architecture, as demonstrated by CNN. Thus, automated lesion detection could potentially improve sensitivity for detecting bone metastases [8,9].

However, the field of AI has progressed rapidly in recent years, and the application of AI in spinal metastasis detection remains nascent. The objective of this article is to review the various AI models utilizing multimodal imaging techniques to detect spinal metastasis.

2. Materials and Methods

2.1. Ethical Review

Ethical review and approval were waived for this study due to it being a systematic review of previously published data and did not involve human participants or the collection of new data.

2.2. Search Strategy

We searched PubMed, Scopus, Web of Science Advance, Cochrane, and Embase (Ovid) databases to identify relevant studies, using a search query with specific keywords like 'spine metastases', 'artificial intelligence', 'machine learning', 'deep learning', and 'diagnosis' (Supplementary Table S1). The population under consideration included adults. The objective was to identify studies reporting the use of AI/DL models in predicting diagnosis and image analysis in spine metastases.

Irrelevant articles, such as studies unrelated to spinal metastases and those purely investigating primary spinal tumors, were excluded. Animal studies, reviews, and non-original research articles were also excluded from our analysis to ensure the inclusion of primary research data relevant to our objective. The electronic search ranged from the period's earliest available date up to 27 January 2025 [8].

2.3. Screening of Studies

Each study's title and abstract were screened for relevance before proceeding to full-text screening, which was independently assessed by two reviewers (P.G. and V.S.). Any discrepancies were addressed through consultation with a third reviewer (S.H.). The screening of studies adhered to the PRISMA (Preferred Reporting Items for Systematic Reviews and Meta-Analyses) guidelines (Figure 1).

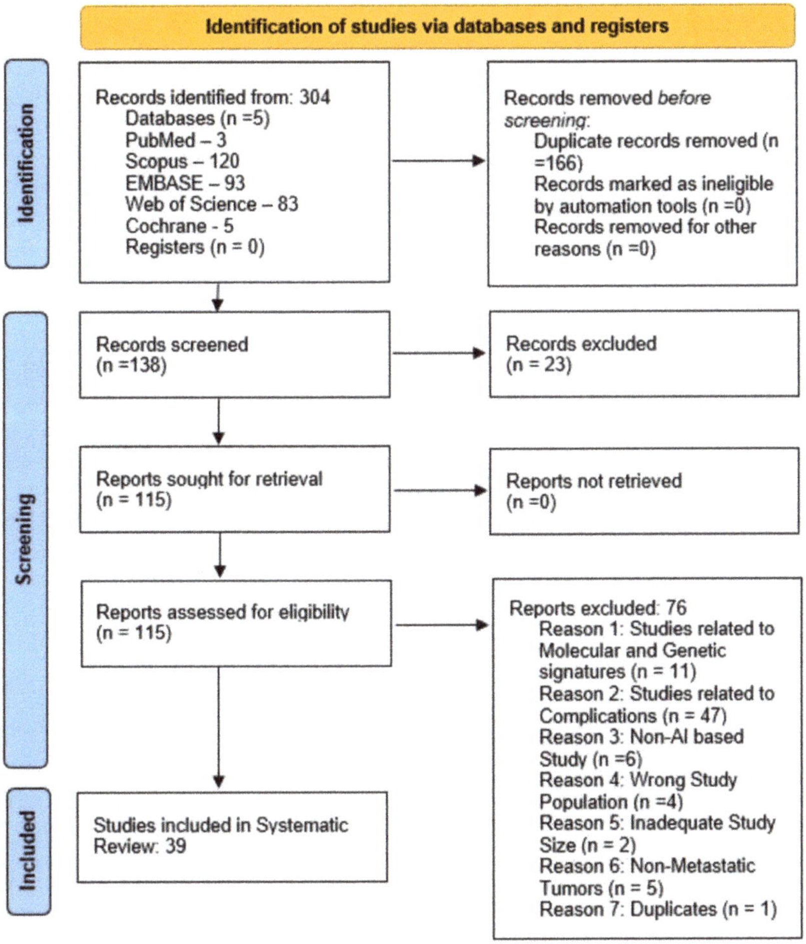

Figure 1. PRISMA flow diagram. A PRISMA flow diagram is presented to illustrate the screening of studies leading to 39 studies being included in the systematic review.

2.4. Data Extraction

Three independent authors (P.G., V.S., and A.T.) extracted relevant data from the included studies. The data collected included study design, participant demographics, and the number of participants with respective outcomes and complications. Discrepancies in data extraction were resolved through consensus [8].

2.5. Data Analysis

Relevant variables were extracted from each of the included articles such as the primary tumor type, cohort size, prediction model performance matrices—area under the receiver operating characteristic curve (AUC)—and type of validation (internal or external validation). The weighted average of the AUC was calculated. All statistical analyses were conducted using Excel, R Statistical Software, version 4.3.1, and Python, version 3.13.3.

2.6. Quality Assessment

The quality assessment was performed using the PROBAST (Prediction model Risk of Bias Assessment Tool (Figure 3 and Figure 4).

PROBAST is designed for assessing the risk of bias and applicability in studies that develop, validate, or update predictive models. It is a structured tool that assesses four domains:

Participants: Evaluating whether the data sources or patient samples used for training and testing are appropriate and representative of the clinical population. Predictors: Ensuring that input data or predictors are well defined and appropriately measured. Outcome: Ensuring that the outcomes (e.g., model predictions, decisions) are clearly defined and relevant to clinical scenarios. Analysis: Evaluating whether the model performance metrics, training/validation processes, and statistical analysis methods are robust and unbiased.

3. Results

This review encompasses 39 studies published between 2007 and 2024, including a total of 6267 patients with a median of 88 patients per study, ranging from 3 to 941 patients. Model performance metrics included AUC, accuracy, sensitivity, specificity, internal validation, and external validation. AUC was most commonly reported, which is why we focused our analysis on that. Out of the 39 studies, 9 reported the number of lesions observed in their study cohorts, with a median of 137 lesions per study. Out of the 39 studies, 12 reported the number of scans performed, with a median of 405.5 scans per study (Table 1).

Table 1. An overview of the studies analyzed is presented, showcasing a set of heterogeneous studies published between 2007 and 2024.

Year of publishing (range)	2007–2024
Total number of patients	6267
Median number of patients	88
Number of patients per study (range)	3–941
Median number of lesions	137
Median number of scans	405.5

Among the 39 studies, the three most common primary tumor types were lung cancer, breast cancer, and prostate cancer, as reported in 22 (56.4%), 20 (51.3%), and 16 (41.0%) studies, respectively (Table 2 and Figure 2). In contrast, neuroendocrine tumors, bladder cancer, and sarcoma were the least common, each reported in two (5.1%), three (7.7%), and three (7.7%) studies, respectively (Table 2). In addition, we also analyzed the primary data modalities used to train and validate the AI models across all 39 studies. Out of the 39 studies included in our systematic review, 20 studies (51.3%) used magnetic resonance imaging (MRI) as the primary data source for their models. In comparison, 17 studies (43.6%) utilized computed tomography (CT), whereas the two remaining studies were based on non-imaging data, such as clinical text for a large language model (LLM) or clinical variables for survival prediction [10,11].

Table 2. The frequency of primary tumor types is shown. Lung cancer proved to be the most common type of cancer analyzed, whereas neuroendocrine tumors were the least common.

Primary Tumor Type	Number of Studies (Percentage)
Lung cancer	22/39 (56.4%)
Breast cancer	20/39 (51.3%)
Prostate cancer	16/39 (41.0%)
Bladder cancer	3/39 (7.7%)
Sarcoma	3/39 (7.7%)
Neuroendocrine tumors	2/39 (5.1%)

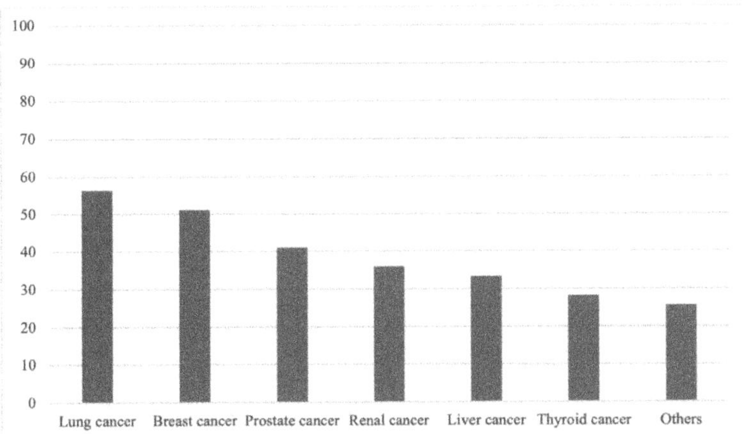

Figure 2. Percentage of studies featuring primary tumor types. The percentage of how many studies feature specific primary tumor types is presented. A wide variety of different cancer types were analyzed in the studies included with lung cancer and breast cancer being represented most often.

Among the 39 studies, 4 reported AUC values for the established models from the training of the model (Table 3), 16 reported AUC values for the established models from an internal validation (Table 4) and five studies reported AUC values from an external validation (Table 5).

Table 3. The AUC (training of each study's best model) and corresponding 95% confidence interval of studies reporting AUC values for the established radiomics models for the training of the model is presented. Three of four studies yielded an AUC of >0.93. [1] = Magnetic resonance imaging.

Study	Output/Prediction	Best Performing Model	AUC	95% CI
Wang et al. (2024) [12]	Prediction of vertebral volumetric bone mineral density in spinal metastases	Deep learning (3DResUNet)	0.977	0.970–0.984
Duan et al. (2023) [13]	Identification of origin for spinal metastases from MRI [1]	Deep learning	0.94	-

Table 3. *Cont.*

Study	Output/Prediction	Best Performing Model	AUC	95% CI
Zhang et al. (2023) [14]	Differentiating spinal metastases from multiple myeloma	Radiomics nomogram	0.856	0.804–0.907
Liu et al. (2022) [15]	Differentiating spinal metastases from multiple myeloma	Radiomics (2EPV-CFS-model)	0.94	-

Table 4. The AUC (internal validation of each study's best model) and corresponding 95% confidence interval of studies reporting AUC values for the established radiomics models for the internal validation of the model is presented. AUCs range from 0.76 to 1.00. [1] = split sample internal validation, [2] = k-fold cross validation, [3] = Computer tomography, [4] = Bagging combined with a REPTree.

Study	Output/Prediction	Best Performing Model	AUC	95% CI
Ahn et al. (2024) [16]	Uncertainty quantification in automated detection of vertebral metastasis	Ensemble Monte Carlo dropout (EMCD; deep learning model)	0.93 [1]	-
Wang et al. (2024) [12]	Prediction of vertebral volumetric bone mineral density in spinal metastases	Deep learning (3DResUNet)	0.966 [1]	0.944–0.988 [1]
Duan et al. (2023) [13]	Identification of origin for spinal metastases from MRI [1]	Deep learning	0.76 [2]	-
Duan et al. (2023) [17]	Differentiating spinal tuberculosis and spinal metastases	Multiscale vision transformers V2 (MVITV2)	0.98 [2]	-
Koike et al. (2023) [18]	Detection and classification of lytic-dominant lesions	Deep learning-based computer-aided detection system	0.941 [1]	-
Li et al. (2023) [19]	Differentiating solitary metastasis and solitary primary tumor	Radiomics nomogram	0.980 [2] 0.924 [1]	0.959–0.995 [2] 0.693–0.916 [1]
Liu et al. (2023) [20]	Prediction of primary tumor sites in spinal metastases	ResNet-50 CNN (deep learning)	0.77 [2]	-
Shi et al. (2023) [21]	Differentiating spinal osteolytic metastases from multiple myeloma	XGBoost with multiparameter DECT (mpDECT)	1.00 [2] 0.97 [1]	- -
Zhang et al. (2023) [14]	Differentiating spinal metastases from multiple myeloma	Radiomics nomogram	0.853 [1]	0.764–0.919 [1]
Chen et al. (2022) [22]	Differentiating spinal metastases from multiple myeloma	Multi-view attention-guided network (MAGN; deep learning Model)	0.785 [2]	0.682–0.888 [2]
Liu et al. (2022) [15]	Differentiating spinal metastases from multiple myeloma	Radiomics (5EPV-16-model)	0.85 [2]	-
Liu et al. (2022) [23]	Differentiating osteolytic from osteoblastic spinal metastases	Radiomics	0.82 [2]	0.71–0.93 [2]
Netherton et al. (2022) [24]	Automating treatment planning for diagnostic and simulation CT [3] scans	Deep learning (U-Net+) and random forest	0.82 [2]	-
Chianca et al. (2021) [25]	Spinal lesion differential diagnosis	Radiomics and machine learning (BaggedREPT [4])	0.90 [1]	-
Filograna et al. (2019) [26]	Identification of most significant predictors of metastasis	Deep learning—logistic regression model (T2-weighted images)	0.912 [2]	0.829–0.994 [2]
Roth et al. (2015) [27]	Detection of sclerotic spine metastases	Deep learning—two-tiered cascade framework	0.834 [2]	-

Table 5. The AUC (external validation of each study's best model) and corresponding 95% confidence interval of studies reporting AUC values for the established radiomics models for the external validation of the model is presented. AUCs range from 0.75 to 0.95. [1] = bagging combined with a REPTree.

Study	Output/Prediction	Best Performing Model	AUC	95% CI
Zijlstra et al. (2024) [11]	90-day survival	Machine learning algorithm (SORG-MLA)	0.81	0.77–0.86
	1-year survival		0.75	0.71–0.80
Duan et al. (2023) [17]	Differentiating spinal tuberculosis and spinal metastases	Multiscale vision transformers V2 (MVITV2)	0.95	-
Duan et al. (2023) [13]	Identification of origin for spinal metastases from MRI [1]	Deep learning	0.76	-
Zhang et al. (2023) [14]	Differentiating spinal metastases from multiple myeloma	Radiomics nomogram	0.762	0.605–0.751
Chianca et al. (2021) [25]	Spinal lesion differential diagnosis	Radiomics and machine learning (BaggedREPT [1])	0.89	-

The weighted average AUC value among the four studies that reported AUC values and the corresponding 95% confidence intervals for the training of the established models is 0.971 (95% CI: 0.965–0.978). Wherever 95% confidence intervals were not reported, the weighted average of the reported 95% confidence intervals was used.

The weighted average AUC value among the 16 studies that reported AUC values and the corresponding 95% confidence intervals for the internal validation of the established models is 0.947 (95% CI: 0.935–0.958). Wherever 95% confidence intervals were not reported, the weighted average of the reported 95% confidence intervals was used.

The weighted average AUC value among the five studies that reported AUC values and the corresponding 95% confidence intervals for the external validation of the established models is 0.819 (95% CI: 0.797–0.840). Wherever the 95% confidence intervals were not reported, the weighted average of the reported 95% confidence intervals was used.

3.1. Risk of Bias Assessment

The risk of bias (Figure 3) and applicability (Figure 4) concerns of the 39 included studies were evaluated using the PROBAST tool, focusing on AI-based predictive models for spinal metastasis diagnosis and image analysis. In the participants domain, 32 studies (82%) demonstrated low risk of bias, with appropriate patient selection and representative cohorts, while five (13%) had high risk and two (5%) had unclear risk, primarily due to the small sample sizes or non-representative populations. For the predictors domain, 28 studies (72%) exhibited low risk with well-defined imaging features, whereas seven (18%) had high risk and four (10%) had unclear risk, often linked to inconsistent feature extraction or unclear predictor definitions. The outcome domain revealed greater variability, with 20 studies (51%) at low risk, 15 (38%) at high risk, and four (10%) at unclear risk; high-risk studies frequently lacked standardized reference standards for metastasis diagnosis or suffered from subjective outcome assessment. The analysis domain presented the most significant concerns, with only 12 studies (31%) at low risk, 22 (56%) at high risk, and five (13%) at unclear risk. Common issues included inadequate external validation, overfitting, and the poor handling of missing data, undermining model reliability and generalizability.

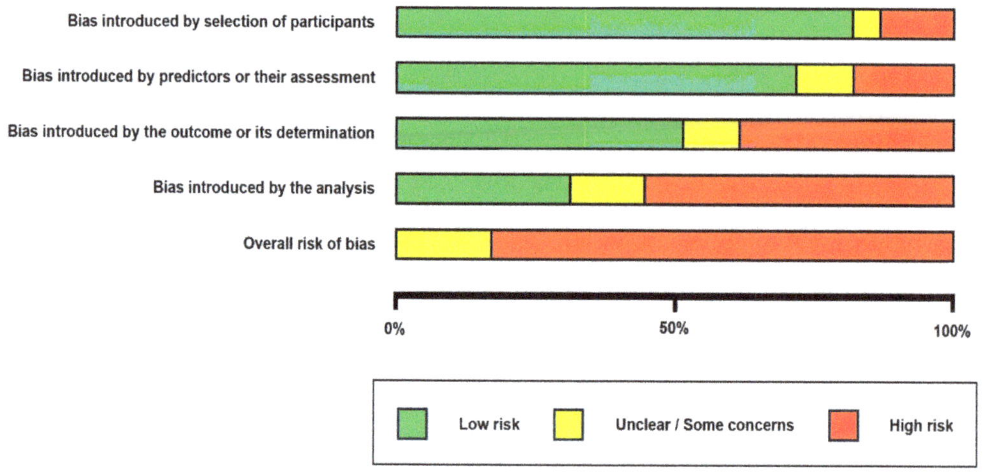

Figure 3. A risk of bias analysis is presented.

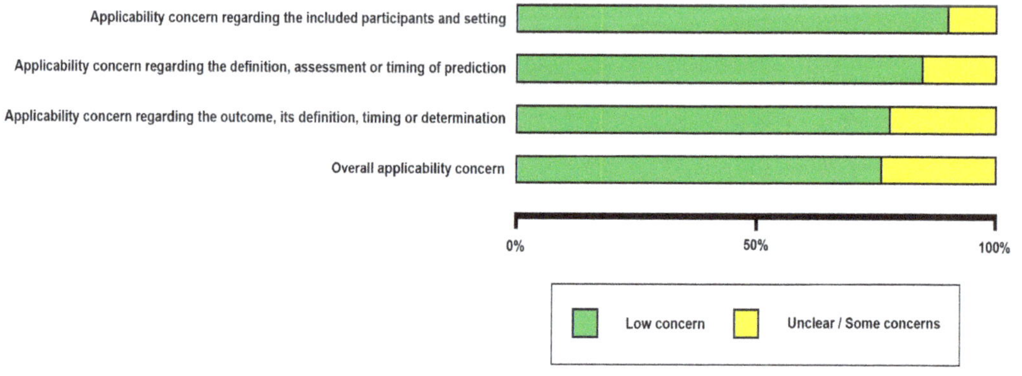

Figure 4. An applicability analysis of the studies included is presented.

Regarding applicability, 35 studies (90%) had low concerns in the participants domain, 33 (85%) in the predictors domain, and 30 (77%) in the outcome domain, indicating relevance to the review's focus on spinal metastasis imaging. However, high applicability concerns in a minority of studies arose from niche cohorts (e.g., specific tumor subtypes) or experimental imaging modalities not widely translatable to clinical practice. Overall, 15 studies (38%) were deemed to have high risk of bias in at least one domain, predominantly the analysis domain, highlighting critical limitations in the current evidence base that may overestimate model performance and warrant the cautious interpretation of reported outcomes.

3.2. Temporal Overview of Included Studies

The 39 included studies were stratified into two temporal groups: those published before 2020 (n = 9) and those published from 2020 onward (n = 30). This analysis revealed a substantial acceleration in research output, with 77% of the studies in this review being published since the beginning of 2020, reflecting rapid advancements in deep learning and computational resources in recent years.

4. Discussion

This systematic review examined 39 studies published between 2007 and 2024, providing a comprehensive evaluation of artificial intelligence applications in spinal metastasis imaging. The findings demonstrate relatively high-performance metrics across various AI methodologies, with weighted average AUC values of 0.971, 0.947, and 0.819 for training, internal validation, and external validation, respectively. These results overall suggest diagnostic potential while highlighting the expected performance drop during validation phases that warrant further consideration. Furthermore, our analysis reveals that deep learning approaches have become increasingly prevalent, with convolutional neural networks (CNNs) and their architectural variants representing the dominant methodologies. This trend aligns with broader developments in medical imaging, where deep learning has demonstrated particular efficacy in semantic segmentation tasks—delineating both vertebral structures and metastatic lesions with precision approaching expert radiologists [28].

Our findings are consistent with a recent meta-analysis, like Papalia et al. [29] and Tao et al. (2025) [30], with the latter reporting pooled sensitivity and specificity values of 0.88 [0.82–0.92] and 0.89 [0.84–0.93], respectively, across AI models for bone metastasis detection [9]. Notably, in this study, deep learning approaches demonstrated a marginally superior performance compared to traditional machine learning methods, with a pooled AUC of 0.95 versus 0.93. This slight performance advantage likely reflects deep learning's capacity for automated feature extraction, potentially capturing subtle imaging biomarkers that may elude conventional radiomic approaches. The relatively consistent performance across different AI architectures suggests that metastatic lesions exhibit reasonably distinctive imaging features that various algorithms can effectively identify. However, we observed variability in model performance between training and validation cohorts (AUC drop from 0.971 to approximately 0.947 (internal validation) and 0.819 (external validation)), which highlights ongoing challenges in developing generalizable models capable of maintaining performance across heterogeneous patient populations and imaging protocols.

The observed performance drop, particularly during external validation (AUC 0.819 versus 0.971 in training) closely mirrors the analytic deficiencies identified by our PROBAST assessment. The high risk of bias in the 'analysis' domain—most notably overfitting, optimistic performance estimates due to inappropriate internal validation techniques, and absent external validation—directly contributes to this degradation. These methodological shortcomings artificially inflate performance during model development, but fail to ensure robustness when tested on new datasets, thus undermining clinical reliability. The discrepancy in validation outcomes therefore reflects not only natural variability, but preventable design limitations. This underscores the importance of rigorous validation practices, including representative external cohorts and transparent reporting, as prerequisites for generalizable AI in spinal metastasis imaging.

Spinal metastasis imaging encompasses multiple modalities, each with distinct advantages. While MRI remains the gold standard with reported sensitivity and specificity exceeding 98% for metastatic lesion detection [31], AI applications span across CT, MRI, PET-CT, and hybrid approaches. Our findings suggest that AI models demonstrate promising performance across these modalities, though direct cross-modality comparisons remain limited by methodological heterogeneity. Another interesting finding in our study is the near-even split in the use of MRI and CT as the primary imaging modalities for AI model development. The slight predominance of MRI-based studies over the widely available CT modality may reflect its superior soft-tissue contrast, critical for assessing tumor characteristics, thereby providing a comprehensive diagnostic picture for clinicians.

Performance variability across different types of lesions merits particular attention. The literature suggests differential performance between osteolytic and osteoblastic metastases, likely reflecting their distinct radiographic presentations [9,23]. Osteolytic lesions typically present with greater contrast against surrounding bone, potentially facilitating more reliable detection compared to the more subtle density changes characteristic of sclerotic metastases [32]. This differential performance has implications for primary tumor-specific applications, given the propensity of certain malignancies [e.g., prostate cancer] toward osteoblastic metastases versus the predominantly osteolytic pattern seen in others [e.g., lung cancer]. Therefore, while the overall diagnostic accuracy reported in reviews like Tao et al. (2025) [30] is high, our findings emphasize that this performance may not be uniform across all metastatic subtypes [30].

Automated systems for lesion detection and characterization may potentially enhance radiologist and clinician performance, particularly for less experienced practitioners by providing a second opinion. Observer studies have demonstrated that AI assistance can significantly improve detection rates, with Ong et al. (2022) reporting improved figure of merit scores for both attending physicians [0.848 to 0.876, $p = 0.01$] and residents [0.752 to 0.799, $p = 0.02$] when assisted by AI algorithms [9]. Another promising application involves reducing false positive rates in metastasis detection. Wang et al. demonstrated a 44.8% reduction in false positives using a Siamese neural network architecture, potentially alleviating a significant challenge in conventional imaging interpretation [33]. This improvement could substantially impact clinical workflow by reducing unnecessary follow-up imaging and interventions prompted by false positive findings. Beyond detection, segmentation represents another valuable clinical application. The accurate delineation of metastatic lesions is crucial for treatment planning, particularly for targeted radiation therapy and minimally invasive interventions. The high dice similarity coefficients reported by Arends et al. [97% and 95% for internal and external validation] show that automated segmentation approaches can produce an impressive performance that warrants direct comparison studies to expert manual segmentation [34]. Such capabilities could significantly improve workflow efficiency while maintaining high accuracy in treatment planning, facilitating the multidisciplinary management of spinal tumors [35]. This shift towards clinically relevant models is a very recent trend, as our temporal analysis confirms: a majority of the included papers were published after 2020. The foundational studies published before 2020 often relied on classical machine learning or computer-aided detection (CAD) systems, which, although pioneering, reflect the technological landscape of an earlier time. In contrast, studies published from 2020 onward predominantly leverage more sophisticated deep learning architectures, which generally report higher diagnostic accuracy and more robust segmentation capabilities. As the field of AI matures rapidly from exploratory concepts to more clinically translatable, high-performance models, these studies are more representative of the current capabilities of AI.

Despite promising results, several challenges currently limit the clinical translation of AI for spinal metastasis imaging. Foremost among these is the persistent gap between training and validation performance metrics, suggesting potential overfitting or limited generalizability. The weighted average AUC decreased from 0.971 during training to 0.947 during internal validation and 0.819 during external validation, highlighting the need for more robust validation approaches and diverse training datasets. Additionally, the pooled AUCs presented in Tables 3–5 need to be interpreted cautiously as they reflect the weighted averages of AUCs of highly varied prediction tasks and thus provide a general overview of AI's current capability of diagnosing spinal metastases, yet they do not allow for significant statements about specific prediction tasks to be made. Furthermore, given the nature of the missing statistical data, wherever 95% confidence intervals were not reported, the weighted average of the reported 95% confidence intervals was used to calculate the weighted average AUC with its corresponding 95% confidence interval. Such imputation may, however, underestimate the true uncertainty of the studies with unreported 95% confidence intervals. This could have led to bias in study weighting, potentially artificially narrowing pooled confidence intervals, especially if the unreported data were from smaller or lower-quality studies.

Data limitations represent another significant challenge. The median cohort size of 88 patients across the reviewed studies indicates relatively modest training datasets by contemporary deep learning standards. This limitation is particularly relevant given the heterogeneity of spinal metastatic disease across the different primary malignancies, imaging protocols, and patient demographics. The predominance of certain primary malignancies in the literature [lung 56.4%, breast 51.3%, prostate 41.0%] may also limit generalizability to less common primary tumors. AI models perform differentially across lesion types. Given that certain kinds of primary tumors tend to give rise to either osteolytic or osteoblastic metastases, the majority of models may have been optimized to detect lesions more commonly found with their respective primary tumor types. Osteolytic metastases (common in lung/breast cancer) show higher detection rates than osteoblastic lesions (typical in prostate cancer), reflecting radiographic contrast differences [36]. This impacts a mixed-dataset training where prostate cancer constituted 41% of studies. This may lead to reduced accuracy in the detection of metastatic lesions with atypical radiographic presentation. Technical challenges in metastasis detection warrant consideration as well. Differentiating metastatic lesions from benign processes such as degenerative changes, hemangiomas, and other non-malignant entities remains challenging even for expert radiologists. While AI may excel at pattern recognition, distinguishing subtle differences between malignant and benign lesions with similar imaging characteristics represents an ongoing challenge.

Several promising directions emerge for future research in this field. First, multimodal approaches integrating complementary information from different imaging sequences [e.g., T1, T2, STIR, diffusion-weighted imaging in MRI] may improve detection sensitivity and specificity. Wallace et al. (2015) highlighted the superiority of multisequence MRI in detecting marrow infiltration before overt trabecular or cortical destruction becomes apparent, suggesting the potential benefits from AI models capable of integrating information across multiple sequences [37]. Second, the integration of clinical data with imaging findings may enhance the overall diagnostic performance. Current AI approaches predominantly focus on image analysis in isolation, neglecting potentially valuable clinical information such as primary tumor characteristics, treatment history, and laboratory parameters. Multimodal models incorporating both imaging and clinical data may better reflect the integrative approach used by clinicians in practice [38]. Third, federated learning approaches represent a promising strategy to address data limitations while preserving patient privacy. Data augmentation techniques have proven effective in bone imaging applications. Various augmentation strategies including geometric transformations (rotation, scaling, flipping), intensity modifications, and elastic deformations have been reported in literature. Advanced augmentation techniques such as generative adversarial networks (GANs) and synthesis-based augmentation have shown promise for creating realistic bone lesion variations while preserving clinical relevance [39]. Multiple studies have successfully employed transfer learning approaches, particularly domain-specific transfer learning within medical imaging. Transfer learning from medical imaging datasets (rather than natural image datasets like ImageNet) can produce significant performance improvements with small training datasets. For bone metastasis detection, transfer learning from related skeletal imaging tasks has shown superior results compared to ImageNet-based initialization [39]. By enabling model training across multiple institutions without centralized data sharing, such approaches could significantly expand the available training data while addressing the privacy concerns inherent in cross-institutional collaboration. Finally, prospective clinical validation studies are essential to demonstrate meaningful clinical impact beyond retrospective performance metrics. Such studies should not only evaluate diagnostic accuracy but also effects on clinical decision making, workflow efficiency, and ultimately patient outcomes.

This systematic review has several strengths, including comprehensive database searches, rigorous methodology following PRISMA guidelines, and a detailed extraction of performance metrics across a diverse range of AI applications. The inclusion of studies spanning nearly two decades provides a robust overview of the evolving landscape of AI in spinal metastasis imaging. However, several limitations warrant consideration. First, the heterogeneity between the included studies complicates direct comparison. The use of a wide range of AI architectures including traditional machine learning, convolutional neural networks, and transformer-based models, imaging modalities such as CT, MRI, and PET, as well as varying validation techniques including split-sample validation and k-fold cross-validation may affect the pooled results. This is because performance metrics are dependent on the underlying model architecture, the nature and quality of the data included, and the rigor of the validation method used. Significant heterogeneity therefore limits the conclusions that can be drawn from the pooled AUCs about specific prediction tasks. This especially holds true when factoring in the second limitation in the form of publication bias, which may have influenced the reported results, with negative or inconclusive studies potentially less likely to be published. Third, the rapid evolution of AI methodologies means that some of the earlier included studies may utilize techniques that are now considered suboptimal compared to state-of-the-art approaches.

5. Conclusions

AI-based approaches show substantial promise for enhancing the detection, segmentation, and characterization of spinal metastatic lesions across multiple imaging modalities. While technical challenges and implementation barriers remain, continued methodological refinements and rigorous clinical validation may soon translate these promising research findings into valuable clinical tools. Future research should focus on developing more generalizable models through larger and more diverse training datasets, integrating clinical and imaging data, multi-institutional data sharing and federated learning, and conducting prospective validation studies to demonstrate meaningful clinical impact.

Supplementary Materials: The following supporting information can be downloaded at https://www.mdpi.com/article/10.3390/jcm14165877/s1, Table S1: Search String; Table S2: Summary of included studies [10–27,32,33,36,40–57].

Author Contributions: Conceptualization, V.S.; Methodology, V.S. and P.G.; Formal Analysis, V.S. and A.T.; Investigation, V.S., P.G., Z.L. and P.H.; Data Curation, V.S. and P.G.; Writing—Original Draft Preparation, V.S.; Writing—Review and Editing, V.S., P.G., A.T., Z.L., P.H., Z.Q., S.H., E.O.R.N., M.J.C., J.R. and A.D.; Supervision, J.R. and A.D.; Project Administration, V.S. All authors have read and agreed to the published version of the manuscript.

Funding: This research received no external funding.

Institutional Review Board Statement: Ethical review and approval were waived for this study due it being a systematic review of previously published data and did not involve human participants or the collection of new data.

Informed Consent Statement: Not applicable.

Data Availability Statement: All datasets used for this study are presented in the manuscript and its Supplementary Materials.

Conflicts of Interest: The authors declare no conflicts of interest.

References

1. Witham, T.F.; Khavkin, Y.A.; Gallia, G.L.; Wolinsky, J.P.; Gokaslan, Z.L. Surgery Insight: Current management of epidural spinal cord compression from metastatic spine disease. *Nat. Clin. Pract. Neurol.* **2006**, *2*, 87–94. [CrossRef] [PubMed]
2. Robson, P. Metastatic spinal cord compression: A rare but important complication of cancer. *Clin. Med.* **2014**, *14*, 542–545. [CrossRef]
3. Halabi, S.; Owzar, K. The Importance of Identifying and Validating Prognostic Factors in Oncology. *Semin. Oncol.* **2010**, *37*, e9–e18. [CrossRef]
4. O'Sullivan, G.J. Imaging of bone metastasis: An update. *World J. Radiol.* **2015**, *7*, 202. [CrossRef]
5. Jensen, M.P.; Qiang, Z.; Khan, D.Z.; Stoyanov, D.; Baldeweg, S.E.; Jaunmuktane, Z.; Brandner, S.; Marcus, H.J. Artificial intelligence in histopathological image analysis of central nervous system tumours: A systematic review. *Neuropathol. Appl. Neurobiol.* **2024**, *50*, e12981. [CrossRef]
6. Avanzo, M.; Wei, L.; Stancanello, J.; Vallières, M.; Rao, A.; Morin, O.; Mattonen, S.A.; El Naqa, I. Machine and deep learning methods for radiomics. *Med. Phys.* **2020**, *47*, e185–e202. [CrossRef] [PubMed]
7. Rogers, W.; Thulasi Seetha, S.; Refaee, T.A.G.; Lieverse, R.I.Y.; Granzier, R.W.Y.; Ibrahim, A.; Keek, S.A.; Sanduleanu, S.; Primakov, S.P.; Beuque, M.P.L.; et al. Radiomics: From qualitative to quantitative imaging. *Br. J. Radiol.* **2020**, *93*, 20190948. [CrossRef]
8. Sanker, V.; Sanikommu, S.; Thaller, A.; Li, Z.; Heesen, P.; Hariharan, S.; Nordin, E.O.R.; Cavagnaro, M.J.; Ratliff, J.; Desai, A. Artificial Intelligence for Non-Invasive Prediction of Molecular Signatures in Spinal Metastases: A Systematic Review. *Bioengineering* **2025**, *12*, 8. [CrossRef]
9. Ong, W.; Zhu, L.; Zhang, W.; Kuah, T.; Lim, D.S.W.; Low, X.Z.; Thian, Y.L.; Teo, E.C.; Tan, J.H.; Kumar, N.; et al. Application of Artificial Intelligence Methods for Imaging of Spinal Metastasis. *Cancers* **2022**, *14*, 4025. [CrossRef]
10. Heisinger, S.; Salzmann, S.N.; Senker, W.; Aspalter, S.; Oberndorfer, J.; Matzner, M.P.; Stienen, M.N.; Motov, S.; Huber, D.; Grohs, J.G. ChatGPT's Performance in Spinal Metastasis Cases—Can We Discuss Our Complex Cases with ChatGPT? *J. Clin. Med.* **2024**, *13*, 7864. [CrossRef] [PubMed]
11. Zijlstra, H.; Kuijten, R.H.; Bhimavarapu, A.V.; Lans, A.; Cross, R.E.; Alnasser, A.; Karhade, A.V.; Verlaan, J.-J.; Groot, O.Q.; Schwab, J.H. Temporal validation of the SORG 90-Day and 1-Year machine learning algorithms for survival of patients with spinal metastatic disease. *Eur. Spine J.* 2024; *online ahead of print*.
12. Wang, Z.; Tan, Y.; Zeng, K.; Tan, H.; Xiao, P.; Su, G. Bone density measurement in patients with spinal metastatic tumors using chest quantitative CT deep learning model. *J. Bone Oncol.* **2024**, *49*, 100641. [CrossRef]
13. Duan, S.; Cao, G.; Hua, Y.; Hu, J.; Zheng, Y.; Wu, F.; Xu, S.; Rong, T.; Liu, B. Identification of Origin for Spinal Metastases from MR Images: Comparison Between Radiomics and Deep Learning Methods. *World Neurosurg.* **2023**, *175*, e823–e831. [CrossRef] [PubMed]
14. Zhang, S.; Liu, M.; Li, S.; Cui, J.; Zhang, G.; Wang, X. An MRI-based radiomics nomogram for differentiating spinal metastases from multiple myeloma. *Cancer Imaging* **2023**, *23*, 72. [CrossRef]
15. Liu, J.; Guo, W.; Zeng, P.; Geng, Y.; Liu, Y.; Ouyang, H.; Lang, N.; Yuan, H. Vertebral MRI-based radiomics model to differentiate multiple myeloma from metastases: Influence of features number on logistic regression model performance. *Eur. Radiol.* **2022**, *32*, 572–581. [CrossRef]
16. Ahn, S.H.; Baek, S.; Park, J.; Kim, J.; Rhee, H.; Chung, Y.E.; Kim, H.; Lee, Y.H. Uncertainty Quantification in Automated Detection of Vertebral Metastasis Using Ensemble Monte Carlo Dropout. *J. Imaging Inform. Med.* **2024**, 1–16. [CrossRef]
17. Duan, S.; Dong, W.; Hua, Y.; Zheng, Y.; Ren, Z.; Cao, G.; Wu, F.; Rong, T.; Liu, B. Accurate Differentiation of Spinal Tuberculosis and Spinal Metastases Using MR-Based Deep Learning Algorithms. *Infect. Drug Resist.* **2023**, *16*, 4325–4334. [CrossRef]
18. Koike, Y.; Yui, M.; Nakamura, S.; Yoshida, A.; Takegawa, H.; Anetai, Y.; Hirota, K.; Tanigawa, N. Artificial intelligence-aided lytic spinal bone metastasis classification on CT scans. *Int. J. Comput. Assist. Radiol. Surg.* **2023**, *18*, 1867–1874. [CrossRef] [PubMed]
19. Li, S.; Yu, X.; Shi, R.; Zhu, B.; Zhang, R.; Kang, B.; Liu, F.; Zhang, S.; Wang, X. MRI-based radiomics nomogram for differentiation of solitary metastasis and solitary primary tumor in the spine. *BMC Med. Imaging* **2023**, *23*, 29. [CrossRef]
20. Liu, K.; Qin, S.; Ning, J.; Xin, P.; Wang, Q.; Chen, Y.; Zhao, W.; Zhang, E.; Lang, N. Prediction of Primary Tumor Sites in Spinal Metastases Using a ResNet-50 Convolutional Neural Network Based on MRI. *Cancers* **2023**, *15*, 2974. [CrossRef] [PubMed]
21. Shi, J.; Huang, H.; Xu, S.; Du, L.; Zeng, X.; Cao, Y.; Liu, D.; Wang, X.; Zhang, J. XGBoost-based multiparameters from dual-energy computed tomography for the differentiation of multiple myeloma of the spine from vertebral osteolytic metastases. *Eur. Radiol.* **2023**, *33*, 4801–4811. [CrossRef] [PubMed]
22. Chen, K.; Cao, J.; Zhang, X.; Wang, X.; Zhao, X.; Li, Q.; Chen, S.; Wang, P.; Liu, T.; Du, J.; et al. Differentiation between spinal multiple myeloma and metastases originated from lung using multi-view attention-guided network. *Front. Oncol.* **2022**, *12*, 981769. [CrossRef]

23. Liu, K.; Zhang, Y.; Wang, Q.; Chen, Y.; Qin, S.; Xin, P.; Zhao, W.; Zhang, E.; Nie, K.; Lang, N. Differentiation of predominantly osteolytic from osteoblastic spinal metastases based on standard magnetic resonance imaging sequences: A comparison of radiomics model versus semantic features logistic regression model findings. *Quant. Imaging Med. Surg.* **2022**, *12*, 5004–5017. [CrossRef]
24. Netherton, T.J.; Nguyen, C.; Cardenas, C.E.; Chung, C.; Klopp, A.H.; Colbert, L.E.; Rhee, D.J.; Peterson, C.B.; Howell, R.; Balter, P.; et al. An Automated Treatment Planning Framework for Spinal Radiation Therapy and Vertebral-Level Second Check. *Int. J. Radiat. Oncol. Biol. Phys.* **2022**, *114*, 516–528. [CrossRef]
25. Chianca, V.; Cuocolo, R.; Gitto, S.; Albano, D.; Merli, I.; Badalyan, J.; Cortese, M.C.; Messina, C.; Luzzati, A.; Parafioriti, A.; et al. Radiomic Machine Learning Classifiers in Spine Bone Tumors: A Multi-Software, Multi-Scanner Study. *Eur. J. Radiol.* **2021**, *137*, 109586. [CrossRef]
26. Filograna, L.; Lenkowicz, J.; Cellini, F.; Dinapoli, N.; Manfrida, S.; Magarelli, N.; Leone, A.; Colosimo, C.; Valentini, V. Identification of the most significant magnetic resonance imaging (MRI) radiomic features in oncological patients with vertebral bone marrow metastatic disease: A feasibility study. *Radiol. Med.* **2019**, *124*, 50–57. [CrossRef]
27. Roth, H.R.; Yao, J.; Lu, L.; Stieger, J.; Burns, J.E.; Summers, R.M. Detection of Sclerotic Spine Metastases via Random Aggregation of Deep Convolutional Neural Network Classifications. In *Recent Advances in Computational Methods and Clinical Applications for Spine Imaging*; Springer: Berlin/Heidelberg, Germany, 2015; pp. 3–12.
28. Zhou, S.K.; Greenspan, H.; Davatzikos, C.; Duncan, J.S.; Van Ginneken, B.; Madabhushi, A.; Prince, J.L.; Rueckert, D.; Summers, R.M. A Review of Deep Learning in Medical Imaging: Imaging Traits, Technology Trends, Case Studies with Progress Highlights, and Future Promises. *Proc. IEEE* **2021**, *109*, 820–838. [CrossRef] [PubMed]
29. Papalia, G.F.; Brigato, P.; Sisca, L.; Maltese, G.; Faiella, E.; Santucci, D.; Pantano, F.; Vincenzi, B.; Tonini, G.; Papalia, R.; et al. Artificial intelligence in detection, management, and prognosis of bone metastasis: A systematic review. *Cancers* **2024**, *16*, 2700. [CrossRef]
30. Tao, H.; Hui, X.; Zhang, Z.; Zhu, R.; Wang, P.; Zhou, S.; Yang, K. Accuracy of artificial intelligence in detecting tumor bone metastases: A systematic review and meta-analysis. *BMC Cancer* **2025**, *25*, 286. [CrossRef]
31. Shah, L.M.; Salzman, K.L. Imaging of Spinal Metastatic Disease. *Int. J. Surg. Oncol.* **2011**, *2011*, 769753. [CrossRef] [PubMed]
32. Motohashi, M.; Funauchi, Y.; Adachi, T.; Fujioka, T.; Otaka, N.; Kamiko, Y.; Okada, T.; Tateishi, U.; Okawa, A.; Yoshii, T.; et al. A New Deep Learning Algorithm for Detecting Spinal Metastases on Computed Tomography Images. *Spine* **2024**, *49*, 390–397. [CrossRef] [PubMed]
33. Wang, J.; Fang, Z.; Lang, N.; Yuan, H.; Su, M.Y.; Baldi, P. A multi-resolution approach for spinal metastasis detection using deep Siamese neural networks. *Comput. Biol. Med.* **2017**, *84*, 137–146. [CrossRef] [PubMed]
34. Arends, S.R.S.; Savenije, M.H.F.; Eppinga, W.S.C.; van der Velden, J.M.; van den Berg, C.A.T.; Verhoeff, J.J.C. Clinical utility of convolutional neural networks for treatment planning in radiotherapy for spinal metastases. *Phys. Imaging Radiat. Oncol.* **2022**, *21*, 42–47. [CrossRef]
35. Houston, R.; Desai, S.; Takayanagi, A.; Tran, C.Q.; Mortezaei, A.; Oladaskari, A.; Sourani, A.; Siddiqi, I.; Khodayari, B.; Ho, A.; et al. A multidisciplinary update on treatment modalities for metastatic spinal tumors with a surgical emphasis: A literature review and evaluation of the role of artificial intelligence. *Cancers* **2024**, *16*, 2800. [CrossRef] [PubMed]
36. Edelmers, E.; Ņikuļins, A.; Sprūdža, K.L.; Stapulone, P.; Pūce, N.S.; Skrebele, E.; Siņicina, E.E.; Cīrule, V.; Kazuša, A.; Boločko, K. AI-Assisted Detection and Localization of Spinal Metastatic Lesions. *Diagnostics* **2024**, *14*, 2458. [CrossRef] [PubMed]
37. Wallace, A.N.; Greenwood, T.J.; Jennings, J.W. Radiofrequency ablation and vertebral augmentation for palliation of painful spinal metastases. *J. Neurooncol.* **2015**, *124*, 111–118. [CrossRef]
38. Romero, M.; Interian, Y.; Solberg, T.; Valdes, G. Targeted transfer learning to improve performance in small medical physics datasets. *Med. Phys.* **2020**, *47*, 6246–6256. [CrossRef] [PubMed]
39. Alzubaidi, L.; Bai, J.; Al-Sabaawi, A.; Santamaría, J.; Albahri, A.S.; Al-dabbagh, B.S.N.; Fadhel, M.A.; Manoufali, M.; Zhang, J.; Al-Timemy, A.H.; et al. A survey on deep learning tools dealing with data scarcity: Definitions, challenges, solutions, tips, and applications. *J. Big Data* **2023**, *10*, 46. [CrossRef]
40. Chen, H.; Atenafu, E.G.; Zeng, K.L.; Chan, A.; Detsky, J.; Myrehaug, S.; Soliman, H.; Tseng, C.-L.; Sahgal, A.; Maralani, P.J. Magnetic Resonance Imaging Frequency After Stereotactic Body Radiation Therapy for Spine Metastases. *Int. J. Radiat. Oncol. Biol. Phys.* **2024**, *119*, 1413–1421. [CrossRef]
41. Mostafa, E.; Hui, A.; Aasman, B.; Chowdary, K.; Mani, K.; Mardakhaev, E.; Zampolin, R.; Blumfield, E.; Berman, J.; De La Garza Ramos, R.; et al. Development of a natural language processing algorithm for the detection of spinal metastasis based on magnetic resonance imaging reports. *North Am. Spine Soc. J. (NASSJ)* **2024**, *19*, 100513. [CrossRef]
42. Xu, Y.; Meng, C.; Chen, D.; Cao, Y.; Wang, X.; Ji, P. Improved localization and segmentation of spinal bone metastases in MRI with nnUNet radiomics. *J. Bone Oncol.* **2024**, *48*, 100630. [CrossRef]
43. Wang, H.; Xu, S.; Fang, K.B.; Dai, Z.S.; Wei, G.Z.; Chen, L.F. Contrast-enhanced magnetic resonance image segmentation based on improved U-Net and Inception-ResNet in the diagnosis of spinal metastases. *J. Bone Oncol.* **2023**, *42*, 100498. [CrossRef]

44. Wang, D.; Sun, Y.; Tang, X.; Liu, C.; Liu, R. Deep learning-based magnetic resonance imaging of the spine in the diagnosis and physiological evaluation of spinal metastases. *J. Bone Oncol.* **2023**, *40*, 100483. [CrossRef]
45. Hoshiai, S.; Hanaoka, S.; Masumoto, T.; Nomura, Y.; Mori, K.; Okamoto, Y.; Saida, T.; Ishiguro, T.; Sakai, M.; Nakajima, T. Effectiveness of temporal subtraction computed tomography images using deep learning in detecting vertebral bone metastases. *Eur. J. Radiol.* **2022**, *154*, 110445. [CrossRef]
46. Steinhauer, V.; Sergeev, N.I. Radiomics in Breast Cancer: In-Depth Machine Analysis of MR Images of Metastatic Spine Lesion. *Sovrem. Tehnol. Med.* **2022**, *14*, 16. [CrossRef]
47. Chang, C.Y.; Buckless, C.; Yeh, K.J.; Torriani, M. Automated detection and segmentation of sclerotic spinal lesions on body CTs using a deep convolutional neural network. *Skelet. Radiol.* **2022**, *51*, 391–399. [CrossRef]
48. Larhmam, M.A.; Mahmoudi, S.; Drisis, S.; Benjelloun, M. A Texture Analysis Approach for Spine Metastasis Classification in T1 and T2 MRI. In *Bioinformatics and Biomedical Engineering*; Springer: Berlin/Heidelberg, Germany, 2018; pp. 198–211.
49. Fan, X.; Zhang, X.; Zhang, Z.; Jiang, Y. Deep Learning on MRI Images for Diagnosis of Lung Cancer Spinal Bone Metastasis. *Contrast Media Mol. Imaging* **2021**, *2021*, 5294379. [CrossRef] [PubMed]
50. Fan, X.; Zhang, H.; Yin, Y.; Zhang, J.; Yang, M.; Qin, S.; Zhang, X.; Yu, F. Texture Analysis of 18F-FDG PET/CT for Differential Diagnosis Spinal Metastases. *Front. Med.* **2021**, *15*, 7. [CrossRef] [PubMed]
51. Chmelik, J.; Jakubicek, R.; Walek, P.; Jan, J.; Ourednicek, P.; Lambert, L.; Amadori, E.; Gavelli, G. Deep convolutional neural network-based segmentation and classification of difficult to define metastatic spinal lesions in 3D CT data. *Med. Image Anal.* **2018**, *49*, 76–88. [CrossRef] [PubMed]
52. Yao, J.; Burns, J.E.; Sanoria, V.; Summers, R.M. Mixed spine metastasis detection through positron emission tomography/computed tomography synthesis and multiclassifier. *J. Med. Imaging* **2017**, *4*, 024504. [CrossRef]
53. Iwano, S.; Ito, R.; Umakoshi, H.; Karino, T.; Inoue, T.; Li, Y.; Naganawa, S. Thoracic Temporal Subtraction Three Dimensional Computed Tomography (3D-CT): Screening for Vertebral Metastases of Primary Lung Cancers. *PLoS ONE* **2017**, *12*, e0170309. [CrossRef]
54. O'Connor, S.D.; Yao, J.; Summers, R.M. Lytic Metastases in Thoracolumbar Spine: Computer-aided Detection at CT—Preliminary Study. *Radiology* **2007**, *242*, 811–816. [CrossRef]
55. Soltani, Z.; Xu, M.; Radovitzky, R.; Stadelmann, M.A.; Hackney, D.; Alkalay, R.N. CT-based finite element simulating spatial bone damage accumulation predicts metastatic human vertebrae strength and stiffness. *Front. Bioeng. Biotechnol.* **2024**, *12*, 1424553. [CrossRef] [PubMed]
56. Lang, N.; Zhang, Y.; Zhang, E.; Zhang, J.; Chow, D.; Chang, P.; Yu, H.J.; Yuan, H.; Su, M.-Y. Differentiation of spinal metastases originated from lung and other cancers using radiomics and deep learning based on DCE-MRI. *Magn. Reson. Imaging* **2019**, *64*, 4–12. [CrossRef] [PubMed]
57. Netherton, T.J.; Rhee, D.J.; Cardenas, C.E.; Chung, C.; Klopp, A.H.; Peterson, C.B.; Howell, R.M.; Balter, P.A.; Court, L.E. Evaluation of a multiview architecture for automatic vertebral labeling of palliative radiotherapy simulation CT images. *Med. Phys.* **2020**, *47*, 5592–5608. [CrossRef] [PubMed]

MDPI AG
Grosspeteranlage 5
4052 Basel
Switzerland
Tel.: +41 61 683 77 34

Journal of Clinical Medicine Editorial Office
E-mail: jcm@mdpi.com
www.mdpi.com/journal/jcm

www.ingramcontent.com/pod-product-compliance
Lightning Source LLC
Chambersburg PA
CBHW062100220926
51850CB00010B/2834
* 9 7 8 3 7 2 5 8 6 6 6 2 5 *